Essential Facts in Geriatric Medicine

SECOND EDITION

CATHERINE BRACEWELL
Consultant Physician in Geriatric Medicine and General
(Internal) Medicine
Newham University Hospital NHS Trust

ROSAIRE GRAY
Consultant Physician in Geriatric Medicine
General (Internal) Medicine and Cardiology
Whittington Hospital NHS Trust

and

GURCHARAN S RAI
Consultant Physician in Geriatric Medicine
Whittington Hospital NHS Trust

Foreword by
FINBARR MARTIN
Physician and Gerontologist
Guys and St Thomas' Hospitals & King's College, London
President-elect
British Geriatrics Society

Radcliffe Publishing
Oxford • New York

Radcliffe Publishing Ltd
18 Marcham Road
Abingdon
Oxon OX14 1AA
United Kingdom

www.radcliffepublishing.com
Electronic catalogue and worldwide online ordering facility.

First Edition 2005

British Library Cataloguing in Publication Data
A catalogue record for this book is available from the British Library.

ISBN-13: 978 184619 467 2

The paper used for the text pages of this book is FSC certified. FSC (The Forest Stewardship Council) is an international network to promote responsible management of the world's forests.

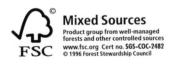

Mixed Sources
Product group from well-managed forests and other controlled sources
www.fsc.org Cert no. SGS-COC-2482
© 1996 Forest Stewardship Council
FSC

Typeset by Pindar NZ, Auckland, New Zealand
Printed and bound by TJI Digital, Padstow, Cornwall, UK

Essential Facts in Geriatric Medicine
SECOND EDITION

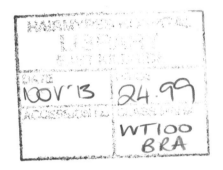

Contents

Foreword

Who amongst us has not panicked at the thought of an exam coming up and just knowing that there are gaping holes in our head where the *essential facts* are meant to be? Where should I turn? What should I read? The massive tome on the library shelf? The web? As tension mounts so the endless expert reviews on the internet search seem, well, . . . endless! But there is another way. For geriatric medicine, be it the College diploma or the specialty examination, this is the book for you.

Geriatric medicine is complex, like our patients. Its breadth encompasses gerontology – social and biological – ethics, law, and virtually the whole of adult medicine. The authors, three highly respected London clinicians, have a wealth of experience in teaching and examining, and it shows. Their book successfully strikes the balance between fascinating detail and core information. It occupies the place between the numerous in-depth specialty texts and the bare bones of core medical training. The scope reflects the syllabus of the specialty-relevant examinations. The depth is a reliable guide to what is needed clinically and what is expected by examiners. The format lends itself to dipping quickly into a chosen topic and also to memorising *essential facts*.

Much of the content, and especially those sections on demography, health and social services and clinical governance, will be of value to all the multidisciplinary team. Likewise the chapters on the legal and ethical domains of clinical practice are an excellent source for the non-specialist posed with new challenges. The authors know that interest will be aroused and for readers who want more, their lists for further reading are an excellent and realistically focused guide.

And if you're thinking that, like me, your exam days are happily behind you, remember, revalidation looms! Meanwhile, the practising geriatrician's role as teacher also requires easy access to *essential facts* for trainer and trainee alike. This is the mission of this book, and is expertly accomplished by Drs Bracewell, Gray and Rai.

Dr Finbarr Martin
Physician and Gerontologist
Guys and St Thomas' Hospitals & King's College, London
President-elect
British Geriatrics Society
June 2010

Preface to the second edition

In writing a new edition of this text, we have not only updated the pre-existing material, but have taken the opportunity to incorporate a number of new subject areas, making it also suitable for trainees in Geriatric Medicine who are preparing for the Specialty Certificate Examination.

The 14 new chapters focus on dizziness, elder abuse, alcohol and drug abuse, HIV in older people, MRSA and clostridium difficile, common skin rashes and skin cancers, renal failure, thyroid disorders, anaemia and haematological disorders, cardiac arrhythmias, osteoarthritis and musculoskeletal disorders, orthogeriatric services, NHS structure and management, and NICE and HAS.

While the main aim of this book is to provide clinical knowledge for doctors preparing for the written examination of the Diploma in Geriatric Medicine and the Specialty Certificate Examination, it should prove valuable to all clinicians including specialist nurses involved in providing care to older people, and medical students.

Catherine Bracewell
Rosaire Gray
Gurcharan S Rai
June 2010

Preface to the first edition

Demographic changes have led to an increasing number of older people presenting to family doctors and hospitals. The healthcare needs of these older people differ substantially from those of younger patients; older patients are more likely to have complex needs in view of the physical, psychological and social changes associated with ageing. In addition, presentation of illness may alter with ageing, as may the response to treatment.

The Royal College of Physicians (RCP) has developed an examination for a Diploma in Geriatric Medicine. The aim is to assess the knowledge and competence of doctors providing care to older people in general practice, of clinicians with an interest in or responsibilities for the care of older people, and of those working in departments of geriatric medicine in non-consultant grades.

Although this book is based on the syllabus for the written examination for the Diploma in Geriatric Medicine, it should prove valuable in every clinical practice and as a useful resource for junior doctors and medical students.

Catherine Bracewell
Rosaire Gray
Gurcharan S Rai
October 2004

About the authors

Dr Catherine Bracewell is a Consultant Physician in Geriatric Medicine and General (Internal) Medicine at Newham University Hospital NHS Trust. She has a keen interest in education and training and has held the roles of Foundation Programme Director and Lead for Care of the Elderly teaching locally.

Dr Rosaire Gray is a Consultant Physician in Geriatric Medicine, General (Internal) Medicine and Cardiology at the Whittington Hospital NHS Trust. She is actively involved in teaching and training of junior medical staff and undergraduates, and research. Her subspecialty areas of interest include stroke and syncope/falls.

Dr Gurcharan S Rai is a Consultant Physician in Geriatric Medicine at the Whittington Hospital. Since his appointment as Consultant Physician he has been actively involved in teaching and training of undergraduates and postgraduates, including those on general professional vocational training schemes, and at the present time he is chairman of the training committee in geriatric medicine in North Thames (East).

Dr Rhodri Edwards is a Specialist Registrar in Geriatric Medicine and General Internal Medicine, University College London Hospital, London.

Abbreviations

AA	attendance allowance
ACE-I	angiotensin-converting enzyme inhibitor
ACTH	adrenocorticotropic hormone
AD	Alzheimer's disease
ADL	activity of daily living
AF	atrial fibrillation
AMPH	approved mental health practitioner
AMTS	abbreviated mental test score
APTT	activated partial thromboplastin time
bd	twice daily
BGS	British Geriatrics Society
BM	blood glucose measurement
BMA	British Medical Association
BMD	bone mineral density
BNP	B-type natriuretic peptide
BP	blood pressure
BPH	benign prostatic hypertrophy
BTS	British Thoracic Society
CA	carer's allowance
CAP	community-acquired pneumonia
CBT	cognitive behavioural therapy
CGA	comprehensive geriatric assessment
CHD	coronary heart disease
CLL	chronic lymphatic leukaemia
CNS	central nervous system
COPD	chronic obstructive pulmonary disease
CPR	cardiopulmonary resuscitation
CSA	Care Standards Act
CSF	cerebrospinal fluid
CT	computed tomography
DBP	diastolic blood pressure
DC	direct current
DEXA	dual energy X-ray absorptiometry
DM	diabetes mellitus
DNAR	do not attempt resuscitation
DVLA	Driver and Vehicle Licensing Agency
ECG	electrocardiograph
ENT	ear, nose and throat
ESR	erythrocyte sedimentation rate
FBC	full blood count
FEV_1	forced expiratory volume in one second

FSH	follicle stimulating hormone
FVC	forced vital capacity
GFR	glomerular filtration rate
GH	growth hormone
GI	gastrointestinal
GMC	General Medical Council
HAS	health advisory service
HIV	human immunodeficiency virus
HONK	hyperosmolar nonketotic coma
HRT	hormone replacement therapy
ICP	intracranial pressure
IGF-1	insulin-like growth factor-1
IHD	ischaemic heart disease
IMCA	independent mental capacity advocate
INR	international normalised ratio
ISH	isolated systolic hypertension
kPa	kilopascal
LA	local authority
LACI	lacunar infarct
LBM	lean body mass
LFT	liver function test
LH	luteinising hormone
LPA	lasting power of attorney
LTOT	long-term oxygen therapy
MAO-B	monoamine-oxidase type B
MCA	middle cerebral artery
MCA 2005	Mental Capacity Act 2005
MCS	microscopy, culture and sensitivity
MCV	mean corpuscular volume
MI	myocardial infarction
MIND	National Association for Mental Health
MMSE	mini-mental state examination
MRC	Medical Research Council
MRI	magnetic resonance imaging
MHRT	Mental Health Review Tribunal
MRSA	methicillin-resistant *Staphylococcus aureus*
NHS QIS	National Health Service and Quality Improvement Scotland
NICE	National Institute for Clinical Excellence
NMDA	N-methyl-D-aspartate
NREM	non-rapid eye movement
NRT	nicotine replacement therapy
NSAID	non-steroidal anti-inflammatory drug
NSF	National Service Framework
NTO	National Training Organisation
NVQ	National Vocational Qualification
OA	osteoarthritis
OCP	ova, cysts and parasites
od	once daily
OPG	Office of the Public Guardian
PACI	partial anterior circulation infarction
PCT	primary care trust
POCI	posterior circulation infarction

PPI	proton pump inhibitor
PSA	prostate-specific antigen
PTH	parathyroid hormone
qds	four times a day
RCT	randomised controlled trial
REM	rapid eye movement
RLS	restless legs syndrome
RNIB	Royal National Institute for the Blind
SaO_2	oxygen saturations
SBP	systolic blood pressure
SSD	Social Services Department
SSRIs	selective serotonin reuptake inhibitors
SNRIs	serotonin norepinephrine reuptake inhibitors
STN-DBS	deep-brain stimulation
T3	triiodothyronine
T4	thyroxine
TACI	total anterior circulation infarction
tds	three times a day
TENS	transcutaneous electrical nerve stimulation
TIA	transient ischaemic attack
TRH	thyrotropin releasing hormone
TSH	thyroid stimulating hormone
TURP	transurethral resection of the prostate
U+E	urea and electrolytes
UKCC	United Kingdom Care Commission
UKPDS	United Kingdom Prospective Diabetes Study
WHO	World Health Organization

PART I

Demographic and social factors

CHAPTER 1

Demography of the ageing population of the United Kingdom

BACKGROUND

- ➤ People are living longer.
- ➤ Birth rates are falling.
- ➤ A global shift in the age structure of populations is occurring with more people than ever aged over 65 years.
- ➤ This age shift has important health, social and economic consequences.
- ➤ Policies to enhance the health, independence and productivity of older people are vital.

AGE STRUCTURE OF THE POPULATION

- ➤ The population of the UK was 58 789 194 according to the 2001 Census.
- ➤ Of this total, 18.4% were over pensionable age.
- ➤ Ethnic minority elders comprise approximately 7% of the population.
- ➤ Similar age shifts are occurring in other First World nations and in developing countries.
- ➤ The world's older population (over 65 years) is growing at a rate of 2.4% annually.
- ➤ In developed countries there are 165 million older people – this is expected to increase to 257 million by 2025.
- ➤ Sweden has the highest number of older people of the major countries of the world (17%) closely followed by the UK, Italy, Belgium and France (16%).
- ➤ The fastest growing segment of the older population is the 'old old' (over 80 years).

FUTURE PATTERNS OF AGEING

- ➤ Life expectancy is increasing with each generation: in 1999 it was 19.2 years for a man aged 60 and 22.8 years for a 60-year-old woman.
- ➤ By 2036 it is estimated that:
  — the number of 60–74 year olds will increase by 50%
  — the over-75 year age group will have increased by 70%
  — the 15–44 age group will have declined by 8%.
- ➤ The number of centenarians in England and Wales is increasing with time:
  — 1951: 300
  — 1996: 5 523 (4 943 women/580 men)
  — 2036: 39 000
  — 2066: 95 000.

FACTORS INFLUENCING AGEING PATTERNS AND TRENDS

➤ Low fertility rates (nearly all developed countries now have fertility rates below the natural replacement level of 2.1 children per woman).
➤ The post-war 'baby boom' will contribute to the accelerated growth of the older population in the second and third decades of the twenty-first century.
➤ Improving mortality rates.
➤ Increasing longevity.
➤ Medical treatment advances and improved health.
➤ Migration.

IMPLICATIONS OF AN AGEING POPULATION ON SOCIETY

➤ The age shift is far-reaching in its implications for healthcare, social support and the economy.

Healthcare

➤ Disabilities and multiple health problems are more common in older people.
➤ Demands on the healthcare service will increase as the population ages.
➤ The World Health Organization (WHO) warns that the health impact of ageing could be enormous and predicts a large rise in cancer, ischaemic heart disease (IHD), diabetes mellitus (DM), dementia and other illnesses relating to old age.
➤ Older people attend emergency departments more frequently than younger people.
➤ Inpatient length of stay is greater for the older person.
➤ GP home visits are most commonly to older people.

Social support

➤ A large proportion of home care services are dedicated to older people.
➤ A growing number of frail older people will necessitate the expansion of social service support for community dwellers and the number of places in residential and nursing care facilities.
➤ Smaller families, more women entering the workforce and younger family members migrating away from the home will mean that fewer people will be available to care for older people when they need assistance.

Economic consequences

➤ More funding will be required, not just to augment health and social services, but to tackle other issues including employment, pensions, transport and town planning.

PLANNING FOR THE AGE SHIFT

➤ The challenges of population ageing are global, national and local.
➤ It is important to understand demographic trends to plan for the future.
➤ People without disabilities face fewer impediments to continued work, use less medical care and require fewer care-giving services.
➤ It is far less costly to prevent disease than to treat it.
➤ WHO has launched a campaign to promote good health in old age and has adopted the term 'active ageing': the process of optimising opportunities for physical, social and mental well-being throughout the life course, in order to extend healthy life expectancy, productivity and quality of life in older age.[1]
➤ The aims of 'active ageing' are to:
　— reduce the number of adults dying prematurely in the highly productive stages of life
　— reduce the number of disabilities associated with chronic diseases

— ensure that older people remain independent and enjoy a positive quality of life
— encourage older people to continue to make a productive contribution to the economy
— reduce the numbers that will need costly medical and care services.
➤ Health promotion should be a top priority for policymakers.
➤ Information and education to promote healthy ageing across the course of people's lives from an early stage should be developed and disseminated as widely as possible.
➤ Policies and programmes need to be put in place to help halt the massive expansion of chronic disease.
➤ Need to focus on health promotion, disease prevention and increasing productivity.
➤ Need to support activities in early life that will enhance growth and development and prevent disease, e.g. obesity, osteoporosis, smoking.
➤ In adult life interventions are needed to prevent, reverse or slow down the onset of disease.
➤ In later life need to focus on maintaining independence, preventing and delaying disease and improving the quality of life for older people who live with some degree of illness or disability.
➤ Need to promote:
— *Physical activity*
  i   Regular, moderate exercise can delay functional decline and reduce the risk of chronic diseases in both healthy and chronically ill older people.
  ii It improves mental health and often promotes social contacts.
  iii Being active can help older people maintain their activities of daily living as independently as possible for the longest period of time.
  iv There are economic benefits: medical costs are substantially lower.
— *Healthy eating*
  i   Malnutrition in older adults includes both under-nutrition and excess calorie consumption.
  ii Obesity and a diet high in fat are related to conditions including cardiovascular disease and osteoarthritis.
  iii Insufficient calcium and vitamin D intake is associated with a loss of bone density and consequently fractures.
— *Tobacco use*
  i   It is never too late to stop smoking.
  ii Even in old age smoking cessation can reduce the rates of IHD, stroke and lung cancer.
— *Alcohol*
  i   Older people are susceptible to alcohol-related diseases as well as being at risk of falls and injuries, and the potential hazards of mixing alcohol and medication.
➤ The determinants of active ageing:
— *Social factors* – education/literacy/human rights/social support/prevention of violence and abuse
— *Personal factors* – biology/genetics/adaptability
— *Health/social services* – health promotion/disease prevention/long-term care/ primary care
— *Physical environment* – urban and rural settings/housing/injury prevention
— *Economic factors* – income/work/social protection
— *Behavioural factors* – physical activity/healthy eating/cessation of tobacco use/ control of alcohol problems/inappropriate use of medication.

➤ The health sector should:
  — reduce the burden of excess disability
  — reduce the risk factors associated with the causes of major diseases and increase the factors that protect health and well-being throughout the life course
  — develop primary healthcare systems that emphasise health promotion, disease prevention and the provision of cost-effective, equitable and dignified long-term care
  — advocate and collaborate with other sectors such as education, housing and employment to affect positive changes in the broad determinants of healthy active ageing.

REFERENCE

1 World Health Organization. *Active Ageing: a policy framework*. Geneva: World Health Organization; 2002. Available at: http://whqlibdoc.who.int/hq/2002/WHO_NMH_NPH_02.8.pdf (accessed 20 May 2010).

FURTHER READING

Office for National Statistics. 2001 Census Data. www.ons.gov.uk/census/index.html

CHAPTER 2

Social processes in ageing

INTRODUCTION

➤ Roles played by an individual over the life course may include:
  — family roles (being son, daughter, wife, husband)
  — social and community roles – neighbour, friend, etc.
  — work roles.
➤ These roles change throughout life and many decline after middle age. The impact of these changes varies from individual to individual and depends upon:
  — the importance attached to them by the individual
  — the importance attached to them by the society
  — the individual's personality
  — the individual's behaviour pattern
  — the individual's financial circumstances in old age.
➤ The three Rs that are said to define tasks of ageing and are associated with successful old age are:
  1 accepting *reality* about one's capacities in health, social and financial realms
  2 fulfilling *responsibilities* – planning for the survivors and making best choices regarding the remainder of life
  3 exercising *rights* – right to live life as an individual at one's pace, right to privacy, right to respect, right to autonomy.
➤ Despite the shift from extended family to nuclear family through mobility of families, size of housing and tendency for both partners to work, most older people still interact with their family and most have a relative living within travelling distance from them.
➤ On the practical and positive side many older people fulfil an increasingly important role of grandparent through:
  — providing support in times of crisis
  — babysitting
  — providing income/financial support
  — acting as confidant
  — being a surrogate parent.
➤ On the negative side many changes associated with ageing may be experienced as losses. These include:
  — physical changes:
  — impaired vision
  — loss/reduction in hearing
  — decline in physical health.
  — changes in social environment:

- retirement (voluntary or involuntary)
- reduced income
- loss of social status
- loss of social interaction
- loss of personal standing/prestige
- loss of home as a result of reduced income (about 40% of pensioners rely on means-tested benefit, and 50% receive at least three-quarters of their income from state benefits)
- loss of privacy when forced to move into an institution.
— family changes:
  - with urbanisation extended family structure has been replaced by nuclear family
  - loss of family members and friends through death
  - strain on family relationships as a result of changes listed above and as a result of illness/disability.

IMPACT OF SOCIAL CHANGES

➤ Effects of these changes will depend on:
  — individual's roles and habits in relation to members of family and society as a whole
  — individual's health
  — his/her behavioural capacities.
➤ In some, these losses with the prospect of their own death may lead to bereavement and depression, while others may accept changes and achieve inner peace and self-acceptance, learn to tolerate the death of a spouse while developing new relationships, teaching others to live, passing on wisdom and finding a suitable living environment that allows maximum independence.

FAMILY RELATIONSHIPS

➤ Family relationships, which provide an important focus for support to older people, are dependent upon/influenced by:
  — previous closeness and supportiveness – satisfying in those who have had successful and close relationships. These individuals often feel they are successful in discharging an important obligation to a loved one. In others, resentment from the past may surface and lead to friction and psychological pain
  — families being close and supportive – if they have not been, they will not magically become so when parents become old and infirm; in fact, resentment may surface
  — extended family versus nuclear family
  — whether older people themselves have to act as carers to their very old relatives
  — changing role of females in society – a significant number are having to go out to work to support their own families and home
  — health and dependency of an individual older person
  — potential for large inheritance – in this situation rivalry may develop among family members. About 60% of older people over 65 are owner-occupiers
  — sibling position/relationship in a family – a rejected child may attempt to win love and recognition by helping the aged parents or may unconsciously punish them for rejection
  — the parents' needs for assistance increase – as this increases, children's attitudes may shift

— actions/behaviours of an older person, e.g. playing manipulative games, using money to wield power, etc., which may lead to unhappy and angry children.

RELATIONSHIP WITH ONSET OF DISABILITY AND ILLNESS

➤ With onset of illness significant changes in family dynamics can take place, depending on previous family relationships. These include:
  — increased stress/anxiety/tension
  — disruption of usual interaction.

➤ It is estimated that there are 6 million carers in the UK and 2.8 million are over the age of 50. Caring, which in most cases is provided by a female relative, a spouse or a daughter, may lead to stress because of:
  — time, effort and energy involved in care giving
  — strain on job
  — strain on own family
  — loss of self-esteem
  — depression and anger.

➤ In managing illness in an older person, family needs should be taken into consideration. Doctors should:
  — ensure that the family feel they are actively involved
  — provide information about the illness, once the patient has given consent for this
  — provide support and acknowledge their contribution.

PART II

Clinical aspects of old age

CHAPTER 3

Age-associated physiological changes

Cross-sectional studies of ageing show that all physiological processes in general decline/deteriorate with age, although not all individuals will go through these changes at the same rate. Listed below are changes (anatomical and physiological) that have been described in cross-sectional studies and their likely impact.

SKIN
Physical
➤ Fine wrinkling.
➤ Dryness.
➤ Laxity.
➤ Appearance of Campbell de Morgan spots.
➤ Cherry haemangiomas.
➤ Seborrhoeic keratosis.
➤ Greying of hairs due to reduction/loss of melanin from hair follicles.
➤ Brittle, slow-growing nails.

Histological
➤ Atrophy of epidermis.
➤ Fall in number of melanocytes.
➤ Reduction in Langerhans cells.
➤ Dermal fibroblasts.
➤ Loss of papillary dermal collagen.
➤ Thickened blood vessels.
➤ Reduction in mast cells.
➤ Reduction in number and function of sweat glands.
➤ Reduction in number of Pacinian and Meissner's corpuscles.

GASTROINTESTINAL TRACT
The mouth
➤ Decrease in production of saliva.
➤ Impaired muscles of mastication.
➤ Tooth loss.
➤ Decrease in taste buds resulting in decrease in taste sensation.
➤ Decline in sense of smell
➤ Enlargement of tongue.
➤ Atrophic changes in jaw.

➤ Senescent vascular lesions resembling those of hereditary haemorrhagic telangiectasia.

Possible impact of age-related changes. Changes in mastication as a result of dental changes; altered salivation and changes in efficiency of chewing due to muscular changes; impaired sense of smell and taste may lead to reduced food intake. This may be exacerbated by the decreased change in opioid and insulin receptors that influence appetite.

Upper GI tract

➤ Pharyngeal muscle weakness and abnormal relaxation of cricopharyngeal muscle.
➤ Reduced oesophageal peristalsis in the very old.
➤ Impaired relaxation of lower oesophageal sphincter.
➤ Increase in incidence of achlorhydria with age caused by chronic atrophic gastritis.

Small bowel

➤ Shortening and broadening of villi.

Possible impact. Impaired absorption/decreased efficiency in absorption, but this does not lead to clinical deficiencies.

Large bowel

➤ Atrophy of mucosa.
➤ Cell infiltration of lamina propria and mucosa.
➤ Hypertrophy of lamina muscularis mucosa.
➤ Increase in connective tissue.
➤ Atrophy of muscle layer.

Possible impact. Impaired motility/increased transit time with tendency to constipation, particularly in immobile older person.

Liver

Decrease in liver volume – absolute and in relation to bodyweight.
➤ Decrease in liver blood flow.
➤ Fall in liver glycogen and ascorbic acid.

Impact. Decline in hepatic drug metabolism; however, conventional liver function tests do not alter with age.

Gall bladder

➤ Hypertrophy of muscles but elasticity of wall may decrease.

Pancreas

➤ Deposition of amyloid in islets of Langerhans and blood vessels.
➤ Reduction in lipase but no change in amylase or bicarbonate.
➤ Duct hyperplasia.

Possible impact. Impaired fat absorption but not clinically significant.

Kidneys
➤ Reduction in size and weight of kidneys.
➤ Reduction in number and size of nephrons.
➤ Fall in number of glomeruli.
➤ Increase in sclerotic glomeruli.
➤ Loss of lobulation of glomerular tuft with thickening of membrane.
➤ Sclerotic changes in larger vessels.
➤ Degenerative changes in tubules.

Possible impact. Decline in glomerular filtration rate (decrease by 50% between the ages of 45 and 80) and impaired tubular function make an older person more susceptible to go into renal failure with dehydration or during an acute illness; dose of drugs which are primarily excreted by the kidneys may need adjustment in older people.

NB: Renal function as measured by urea and creatinine reveals no abnormality in fit older person.

BLADDER
➤ Increased incidence of trabeculation and pseudodiverticula.
➤ Changes in urethral epithelium to stratified squamous.
➤ Alteration in vascularity of submucosa.
➤ Decline in bladder capacity.
➤ In men there is tendency for prostate gland to enlarge with age.

Possible impact. These changes by themselves do not produce clinical symptoms but increase the likelihood of urinary tract infection developing.

BONE
➤ Bone loss (thinning of trabeculae and enlarged cancellous spaces) due to increased osteoclastic activity.
➤ Reduced ability to maintain matrix integrity.
➤ Fall in circulating hormones, such as growth hormone involved in maintaining tissue integrity.

Impact. Bone mass declines after middle age, with more marked decline during the first 5 years of menopause. By the age of 70, 50% of bone mass is lost in postmenopausal women, primarily due to fall in oestrogen level. Can be asymptomatic or lead to slight backache, kyphosis or stooped posture.

CARTILAGE OF JOINTS
➤ Breakdown of surface of cartilage (thinning, decrease in stiffness predisposing to osteoarthritis [OA]).

HEART
➤ Loss of myocytes in ventricles.
➤ Increase in interstitial fibrosis and collagen lead to increased stiffness of left ventricle.
➤ Deposition of amyloid, primarily in atria.
➤ Thickening of posterior left ventricular wall due to increase in volume.
➤ Increase in left atrial size.
➤ Increased stiffness of ventricles, thickening of the endocardium and valves.

➤ Increase in circulating catecholamines.
➤ Reduction in pacemaker cells in sinus node.

BLOOD VESSELS
➤ Thickening of smooth muscles in arterial wall – dilatation of large elastic arteries.
➤ Increase in systolic blood pressure due to increased stiffness of peripheral vessels and widened pulse pressure – this may impair left ventricular diastolic function.
➤ A slight decrease in diastolic blood pressure after the sixth decade.

Impact. (1) Prolonged myocardial contraction due to slow relaxation; (2) reduction in resting stroke volume and cardiac output; (3) decline in cardiovascular response to stress/exercise.

NB: While systolic function deteriorates on exercise, there is no reduction in resting LV ejection fraction; fourth heart sound may be heard in 60% of normal older people; basal crackles may be present in immobile older person without heart failure; peripheral oedema may occur in immobile older person without heart failure.

RESPIRATORY SYSTEM
➤ Reduction in number of glandular epithelial cells – reduction in production of protective mucosa and impaired defence against infection.
➤ Changes in respiratory muscles – impaired strength and endurance.
➤ Ossification of costal cartilages, calcification of rib articulatory surfaces with muscular changes lead to impaired mobility of thoracic cage – fall in chest wall compliance.
➤ Thinning of alveoli.
➤ Lung volumes: small increase in total lung capacity, large increase in functional residual capacity, fall in vital capacity, FEV1, with a fall in FEV1/FVC to a mean of 65% from age 70 and decline in maximal oxygen uptake.

CENTRAL NERVOUS SYSTEM CHANGES
➤ Reduced brain weight – reduces after age 40–50 by 2–3% per decade.
➤ Brain shrinkage of overlying gyri.
➤ Thickening of meninges.
➤ Decrease in both grey and white matter.
➤ Decline in nerve cell number, the greatest loss occurring in frontal and temporal cortices.
➤ Decrease in synaptic density in some areas.
➤ Plaques containing β amyloid protein – found in over 70% of those over 80 years.
➤ Neurofibrillary tangles particularly in hippocampus and temporal cortex.
➤ Increase in CSF fluid spaces.

Impact. Age-related changes in pupils may be interpreted wrongly as indicating pathology; decreased density of pain receptors in skin – diminished sensitivity to light touch; altered pressure perception for one- or two-point discrimination; change in pain threshold; slowing of nerve conduction; decrease in ability to detect vibratory stimuli in fingers; tendon reflexes may be difficult to elicit and ankle jerk may be absent in normal older person as a result of age-related changes in sensory fibres.

HEARING

➤ Loss of hair cells in the cochlea. Loss of ganglion cells in the cochlea. Decrease in average number of fibres in the cochlear nerve. All these changes lead to presbyacusis, i.e. loss of hearing for high frequency sounds.

EYES

➤ Flatter cornea leading to astigmatism.
➤ Hardening of lens and iris.
➤ Reduced response from ciliary muscles.
➤ Floaters in vitreous humour.
➤ Changes in skin and muscles leading to enophthalmos and ptosis – ptosis of upper eyelid seen in 11% of normal adults over age of 50.
➤ Small pupil – diameter of 1 mm or less commonly found in older persons.
➤ Pupils respond slowly to light.

Impact. Impaired near vision and astigmatism.

LEAN BODY MASS

➤ After the age of 40, lean body mass (LBM) falls, with rate of loss increasing with increasing age.
➤ Loss of number of muscle fibres plus possible reduction in size of remaining fibres and motor neurones.
➤ *Impact.* Reduction in strength which may contribute to development of disability and falls. In addition one may note mild limb rigidity and paratonia.

FAT MASS

➤ Cross-sectional studies show increase in fat mass with age in both men and women; the increase in females is linear through to the eighth decade of life.

AEROBIC CAPACITY

➤ Decreases in sedentary older people at the rate of 10% per decade. This of course can be increased by physical training in older people between the ages of 60 and 80.

BODY TEMPERATURE

➤ Impaired ability to maintain body temperature through thermogenesis.
➤ Impaired sweating, impaired shivering, impaired cutaneous vasoconstriction response to cold.
➤ Impaired perception of change in temperature.
➤ *Impact.* These changes increase the older person's susceptibility to hypothermia.

GLUCOSE HOMEOSTASIS

➤ In older people (60–90 years) insulin level rises sharply and then drops below the young adult mean – this is probably due to reduced sensitivity of muscles to insulin, insulin resistance and fall in insulin receptors in fat cells.
➤ *Impact.* Impaired glucose tolerance test – plasma glucose rises to higher level and may remain elevated for longer. This is associated with a delay in rise of plasma insulin.

HORMONAL CHANGES

➤ *Reduced oestrogens.* Vaginal dryness, thinning of vaginal wall, vaginal shape – these changes may lead to pain and bleeding during coitus. In addition the changes in oestrogen lead to an increase in bone loss with the POTENTIAL to produce osteoporosis.

➤ *Rise in FSH and LH.*

➤ *Adrenocortical function.* Basal, circadian rhythm and response to ACTH stimulation show no change with ageing.

➤ *Growth hormone.* Declines with age from a peak at about 30 years – decline being approximately 15% per decade. Decrease in circulating levels of insulin-like growth factor-I (IGF-I), a mediator through which GH produces its effects.

➤ *Thyroid.* With ageing it is common to find a decrease in size of follicles, progressive fibrosis and infiltration with lymphocytes. However, circulating free T4 and T3 do not change, except during an illness. In the very old, i.e. over 80, thyroid activity may be low because of decrease in TSH and impairment of peripheral 5-deiodination. Impaired release of TSH – impaired TRH stimulation test.

➤ *PTH.* Serum levels rise with age. An older person has 30% higher levels than a young person. This correlates with decrease in vitamin D levels. These changes contribute to the age-related bone loss.

BLOOD

➤ Although there are bone marrow changes and the response of bone marrow to stimulation is reduced, there is little change in circulating cells with ageing.

➤ No change in levels of plasma coagulation factors.

CHANGES IN IMMUNITY

➤ Increased immune deficiency, although variable, occurs and is due to decline in both cell-mediated and humoral immunity (reduction in active peripheral T-cells with increase in immature T-cells).

➤ Reduced T-cell response to interleukins and mitogens, reduction in the generation of cytotoxic T-cells and humoral immunity (reduction in peak antibody response to immunisation and reduction in the duration of antibody response to immunisation).

PSYCHOLOGICAL CHANGES

➤ Slowing of response to stimuli.
➤ Slowing of central processing information, i.e. slow response to cognitive tasks.
➤ Difficulties in developing concepts.
➤ Difficulty in thinking abstractly – better performance on concrete tasks.
➤ Become more rigid/less flexible.
➤ Curtail activities.
➤ Show increased reflectiveness.

Memory

➤ Require more time and effort to encode.
➤ Worsening of recall memory.

Intelligence

➤ While cross-sectional studies suggest a decline with ageing, longitudinal data does not support this. More specifically, performance on verbal testing remains while performance on tests that require speed of response deteriorates with ageing.

PERSONALITY

Four personality types have been identified with ageing.

1 *Integrated individual.* 'Well-functioning', active person with intact cognitive abilities, is good organiser, flexible and satisfied with life. Some of these individuals voluntarily withdraw from role commitments and accept a so-called rocking-chair approach to life – happy with the past and present and having little fear of the future.

2 *Armoured or defended individual.* Tries to fight the process of ageing and accepts each difficulty as a new challenge, but is often preoccupied with losses.

3 *The passive–dependent individual.* These individuals in their younger days were passive and apathetic and in old age have strong dependency needs and low level of life satisfaction. May have wish for death as they do not wish to be a burden.

4 *Angry individual.* This individual shows gross psychological pathology. The low activity and very low life satisfaction this individual experienced in younger days persist in old age and the person may often be bitter because of what they see as inequalities between old age and youth.

STRESS AND COPING

The key factors that appear to have an impact on the individual's ability to cope with stresses associated with ageing as their role changes include financial resources, social and family supports, health, education, personality traits, religious belief and ability to develop specific coping strategies with stresses posed by retirement and bereavement.

CHAPTER 4

Prevention of disease and disability

With increasing survival, many older people can live 15–20 years beyond retirement and therefore prevention of disease is important. Furthermore, the increased level of disease and disability among the very old indicates that ways of preventing problems must be sought and implemented. The overall objective for older people should be to improve 'independent life expectancy'. Prevention may be classified as in Table 4.1.

TABLE 4.1 Classification of prevention

Primary
Prevention of disease occurrence (e.g. health promotion, immunisation)
Secondary
Early detection of disease (e.g. screening for cancers)
Tertiary
Prevention of complications of established disease (e.g. contractures after stroke)

PRIMARY PREVENTION
Health promotion
Health promotion comprises efforts to enhance positive health and prevent ill health through health education, illness prevention and environmental health. Advice on lifestyle modification, such as stopping smoking, better diet and exercise, is valuable for older as well as younger people. Other measures such as retirement training and bereavement counselling may also be important.

Social and economic factors
It is important to protect the living standards and disposable income of older people in order that they have access to healthy choices in lifestyle. Half of pensioner households depend on the state pension for 75% of their income and relative poverty shows a clear association with increased morbidity in terms of the number of chronic conditions and deteriorating functional status. It is important to identify and target disadvantaged groups such as ethnic minorities.

Diet
It is difficult for many older people to obtain an appropriate diet, due to limited income, limited access to transport and personal mobility problems. High prices in local shops, price differentials making 'healthy foods' more expensive and inappropriately packaged foods all contribute to making healthy choices more difficult for older people. Dietary counselling, especially at retirement, is effective in improving people's choice of healthy foods.

Exercise

Regular exercise improves strength, stamina, suppleness and well-being; however, the proportion of people taking regular exercise decreases with age. Regular appropriate exercise is associated with reduced cardiac and cerebrovascular disease, increased bone strength and a reduction in falls. Exercise needs to be continued for the benefits to be maintained. Health centres and local authorities increasingly offer active programmes to encourage the over-50s to take regular exercise. These need to be extended and tailored to meet the needs of the more frail. In order to enjoy the benefits of exercise, some older patients may need chiropody, help with arthritis and pain relief, and reliable transport, and these issues need to be addressed.

Accidents

There is an increasing risk of falls and accidents both in and outside the home with ageing. Poor lighting, environmental and domestic design, and personal factors such as decreasing visual acuity and balance are important factors. Recognised risk factors for recurrent falls include prescribed medication, lower limb disability, dementia and visual impairment. Along with increasing osteoporosis, especially in postmenopausal women, they lead to an increased rate of fractured neck of femur. Multifactorial intervention concentrating on medication adjustment, exercise programmes and adjusting the home environment can reduce the risk by 30%. Vitamin D and calcium supplementation can reduce fracture rates in nursing home patients and hip protectors reduce fracture rates in residential homes. Hormone replacement therapy (HRT) can reduce fracture rates following falls, but at present there are major concerns over the increased risk of breast cancer and cardiovascular and thrombotic disease associated with its use, so it is not currently recommended. The bisphosphonates also reduce fracture rates and are useful in those who can tolerate them.

Immunisation

Influenza and pneumonia cause high levels of morbidity and mortality in older people. Meta-analyses of 20 cohort studies involving 30 000 older patients show that influenza A and B vaccination reduces the risk of pneumonia and hospitalisation by 50% and death by 70%. Cost-benefit analysis in the UK has shown that immunisation should be offered to all people aged 65 and over and a target uptake of 70% has been set. Pneumococcal vaccination has a 50–80% efficacy in preventing pneumococcal bacteraemia in those over 65 years and those with chronic lung disease and heart disease. Vaccination should be offered to these groups and provides protection for 3–5 years.

SECONDARY PREVENTION

Screening is the detection of disease at an early pre-symptomatic stage, before the patient would normally seek medical help. There is good evidence to support screening in older people, but unfortunately policy does not always accord with scientific evidence and older people are often not included in screening programmes. In practice, the benefits are likely to be at least as great, if not greater, among older people than among young people. It is important to recognise the difference between screening and case finding. Screening aims to measure all eligible people, whereas case finding is the opportunistic detection of disease or problems, usually when patients attend the surgery, often with another problem. The cost and ethical aspects of the two approaches are very different. Case finding is relatively cheap and raises few ethical issues. Screening is more expensive and implies that the services are sufficient to deal with all the problems detected. Some examples where screening is beneficial follow.

➤ Treatment of hypertension has been shown to reduce the risk of stroke by up to 75%. As the risk of stroke increases dramatically with age, many more strokes will be prevented by treatment of hypertension in older people, compared to young adults who have a low risk of stroke.

➤ Statins are effective lipid-lowering drugs and recent trials have shown that the beneficial effects in primary and secondary prevention are evident in older patients.

➤ Aspirin and warfarin are beneficial in reducing stroke in patients with atrial fibrillation, but are often not prescribed for older patients in spite of the fact that both conditions are more common in older people.

➤ Despite evidence to support mammography and cervical smear screening in older women, these services are not offered to women over the age of 65, although they can request a test.

➤ The benefits of screening for prostate in the UK remains unclear, but has been endorsed in the US. Screening programmes for colorectal cancer are now available in the UK.

➤ Simple measures for checking visual acuity, screening for glaucoma, hearing, dental and locomotor activity would make a significant contribution to the quality of life of older people if coupled to ease of access to corrective procedures of known effectiveness.

TERTIARY PREVENTION

In many cases this is detecting disease that, although symptomatic, is largely unrecognised or under-reported. Older patients are more likely to have covert problems that are attributed to the ageing process by both patients and health professionals. The 1990 GP Contract required GPs to offer an annual visit to every person over 75 years to assess the following problems:

➤ visual and hearing impairments
➤ immobility
➤ mental conditions (depression and dementia)
➤ physical conditions (incontinence)
➤ use of medications.

All of these problems are common in older people, but there is a significant shortfall in the diagnosis of these disorders. Early detection and treatment of these problems would improve the patient's physical, mental and social well-being. Unfortunately, this screening is no longer required so a valuable opportunity is being missed.

A number of treatments for established disease have been shown to be beneficial in older people. Such areas include hip replacement surgery, treatment of coronary heart disease (CHD), valve replacement, general surgery and anti-cholinesterases in dementia. Unfortunately, many older people still do not have equity of access to these important therapies, which have been shown to improve their quality of life.

CHAPTER 5

Specific features of disease presentation

While an older person as well as a younger person can exhibit clinical features that lead to a unifying single diagnosis, a significant number do not. The differences between these sick old people and younger persons can be summarised by the helpful mnemonic 'NAMES'.

➤ Non-specific presentation.
➤ Atypical or uncommon presentation.
➤ Multiple pathologies or diagnoses.
➤ Erroneous attribution of symptoms to old age.
➤ Single pathology/illness can lead to catastrophic consequences.

NON-SPECIFIC PRESENTATION

The non-specific presentation has been described in terms of 'dragons' by the first President of the British Geriatrics Society, Dr Trevor Howell, and as 'giants of geriatric medicine' by Professor Bernard Isaacs. Recently, geriatricians have tried to fit the pattern of presentation into an aide-memoire using the letter 'I'.

'Dragons'	'Giants of geriatric medicine'	'I's'
Confusion	Confusion	Intellectual failure
Incontinence	Incontinence	Incontinence
Contractures of joint	Immobility	Immobility
Bedsores and other ulcers	Falls	Instability
Falls		Iatrogenic illness

With such non-specific presentation differential diagnosis in a sick older person can be broad and the doctor has to use all available information from the history (which may have to be sought from a third party) and carry out a full examination and appropriate investigations to find the cause of vague symptoms.

ATYPICAL OR UNCOMMON PRESENTATION

Atypical or uncommon symptoms may replace the commonly stated/quoted features of illness, for example:
➤ myocardial infarction, instead of producing central crushing chest pain with radiation into the left arm or the neck, may present with shortness of breath or a fall resulting from a cardiac arrhythmia or hypotension or with confusion

➤ pneumonia or other serious infections may not give rise to an elevated white cell count or rise in temperature
➤ peptic ulcer perforation in an older person can be asymptomatic and may not produce the classic rigid abdomen with rebound tenderness, and the diagnosis may be made by examination of the chest X-ray
➤ psychiatric illness may present with vague physical symptoms or multiple somatic complaints
➤ apathetic thyrotoxicosis, silent pulmonary embolism
➤ heart failure without dyspnoea.

MULTIPLE PATHOLOGIES
With ageing there is an increasing tendency for many pathologies, which increases the risk of iatrogenic illness in old age. The main factors that contribute to the development of multiple diseases in older people include:
1 increase in age-related incidence of common disorders, e.g. hypertension, osteoarthritis, diabetes mellitus, vascular disease, dementia
2 impaired immune system leading to increased chances of cancer and hypothyroidism
3 increased likelihood of an illness affecting one system leading to disorder in another, e.g. respiratory infection leading to development of atrial fibrillation and heart failure
4 vascular diseases may develop gradually and during the latent period acute illness may develop in an older individual
5 immobility associated with many neurological or musculoskeletal disorders may lead to an increased risk of developing complications such as falls, urinary incontinence, infections, pressure sores, deep vein thrombosis plus pulmonary embolism.

ERRONEOUS ATTRIBUTION OF SYMPTOMS IN OLD AGE
Doctors as well as older people themselves may mistakenly attribute non-specific signs and symptoms to old age. It is not uncommon to hear an older person say 'It is my age, doctor' or 'I am only here because my son or daughter is worried'. One of the reasons for an older person not presenting early with symptoms is denial, fear of what might be found.

SINGLE ILLNESS/PATHOLOGY LEADING TO CATASTROPHIC CONSEQUENCES
While in a young person a simple illness (such as an influenza) may produce symptoms that last for a few days, in some older people it can lead to a cascade of events with dire consequences (*see* Figure 5.1).

OTHER CONSEQUENCES OF ILLNESS IN OLD AGE
➤ Apart from abnormality of one or more organs of the body, an illness has other consequences for the individual as a whole, leading to physical, psychological, functional and social problems.
➤ The impairments, disabilities and handicaps associated with the illness in an older person require full and thorough assessments, not only from a physician but from other professionals, whose roles are to develop and implement rehabilitation in order to achieve maximum recovery and function.
➤ If handicap or disability cannot be abolished, then the team tries to ensure that an individual is able to live as independent a life as possible with support

of individuals or aids and adaptations and services that meet their needs (*see* Chapter 7).

➤ In attempting to meet the physical and psychological needs of an individual, professionals try to reduce the individual's distress, improve their well-being and quality of life (people themselves are the best judges of what makes 'life worth living').

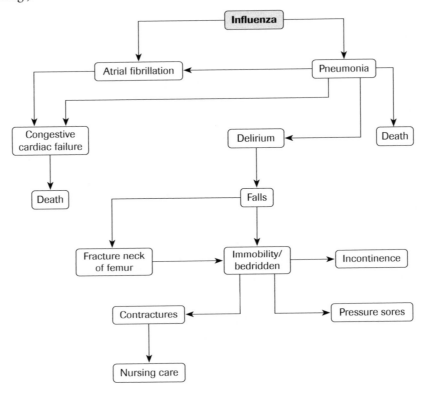

FIGURE 5.1 Potential consequences of a simple illness for older people.

Reproduced from *Elderly Medicine: a training guide*, edited by Gurcharan S Rai and Graham P Mulley. By permission of Martin Dunitz, Andover.

PHYSICAL SIGNS AND OLD AGE

Age-related changes may lead to physical signs or may influence the sensitivity of physical signs in indicating the presence of a disease process. Examples of these include:

➤ small pupils that respond sluggishly to light
➤ changes in eyelids producing ptosis
➤ absent ankle jerks
➤ reduced vibration sensation in fingers
➤ displaced apex beat due to the presence of kyphoscoliosis
➤ presence of pulmonary crackles in the absence of cardiac or pulmonary disease in the immobile older person.

FURTHER READING

Hodkinson HM. Non-specific presentation of illness. *BMJ*. 1973; **4**: 94.

Horan MA. Presentation of disease in old age. In: Tallis RC, Fillit HM, Brocklehurst JC (editors). *Textbook of Geriatric Medicine and Gerontology*. Edinburgh: Churchill Livingstone; 2000. pp. 201–6.

Isaacs B, Livingstone M, Neville Y (editors). *Survival of the Unfittest*. London: Routledge & Kegan Paul; 1972.

CHAPTER 6

Pharmacology and therapeutics

Older people receive more prescriptions per head than any other group.
➤ 45% of NHS prescribing is for people over 65 years of age.
➤ 36% of people aged 75 and over are taking four or more prescription drugs.

Prescribing for older people is complex.
➤ Chronic illness increases with age, so older people are more likely to have conditions that require drug treatment.
➤ There is increasing evidence that primary and secondary prevention therapies benefit older as much as younger patients and this has added to the need for multiple medications.
➤ The hazards of prescribing, including side-effects, adverse drug reactions (ADRs), drug interactions and difficulties of compliance are particularly important in older people.

The Royal College of Physicians report Medication for Older People indicated that excessive prescribing was widespread in older people and recommended careful consideration as to whether drug treatment was appropriate.[1] A list of medication that should be avoided or used with great caution in older people has been published in the United States.[2] The National Service Framework (NSF) for Older People,[3] has set out a series of strategies to improve prescribing including regular medication review, improved communication between primary and secondary care, involvement of pharmacists in prescribing advice and support, patient and carer education to improve compliance and ongoing education and training of staff in health and social care.

Proper use of medication in older people has beneficial effects so older patients should not be denied medication on the basis of age. In the past older patients were often excluded from clinical trials so the applicability of evidence derived from studies in younger patients was often questioned. As more older patients are included in trials the evidence base is increasing but there are still considerable gaps in our knowledge. Even allowing for this, there is evidence that older patients are under-prescribed useful drugs, including aspirin for secondary prevention in high-risk patients, β-blockers following myocardial infarction, and warfarin for nonvalvular atrial fibrillation. There is also evidence that older people receive medications that could potentially cause more harm than good and in particular sedatives and hypnotics. A key difference in distinguishing appropriate from inappropriate drug use is evident in the themes of polymedicine and polypharmacy.
➤ *Polymedicine* describes the use of medications for the treatment of multiple comorbid conditions.
➤ *Polypharmacy* represents a less-than-desirable state with duplicative medications,

drug-to-drug interactions, and inadequate attention to pharmacokinetic and pharmacodynamic principles.

ADVERSE DRUG REACTIONS (ADRs)

Drug related illness is a significant problem in older people. ADRs account for 5–17% of hospital admissions and 6–17% of older patients in hospital experience ADRs.[2] The risk of an ADR increases with age and the number of drugs prescribed. The majority of ADRs are dose related and potentially avoidable. Several mechanisms may account for this including:

➤ Altered pharmacokinetics and pharmacodynamics with age (see below).
➤ Increased sensitivity of diseased tissue to drug toxicity.
➤ Difficulties in patient compliance with an increasing number of drugs.
➤ Prescription of drugs that are unnecessary for the treatment of ailments that might be better managed through non-pharmacological management.
➤ Inappropriate prescription of drugs that are either contraindicated or prescribed in combination with other drugs that produce potential drug interaction.

Drug-drug interactions constitute only a small proportion of ADRs. They are often predictable and therefore avoidable. The most important mechanisms for drug-drug interactions are the inhibition or induction of drug metabolism, and pharmacodynamic potentiation or antagonism. Interactions involving a loss of action of one of the drugs are as frequent as those involving an increased effect. It is likely that only about 10% of potential interactions result in clinically significant events and, while death or serious clinical consequences are rare, low-grade morbidity in older people is more common. Non-specific complaints (e.g. confusion, lethargy, weakness, dizziness, incontinence, depression, falls) should prompt a closer look at the patient's drug list.

Factors affecting drug metabolism include:
➤ Pharmacokinetics.
➤ Pharmacodynamics.
➤ Pharmacogenetics.
➤ Gender.
➤ Frailty and Disease.

Changes in pharmacokinetics and pharmacodynamics with age are listed below and often result in a prolonged drug half-life, increased potential for drug toxicity, and greater likelihood for ADRs.

ALTERATIONS TO PHARMACOKINETICS WITH AGEING

➤ The absorption of drugs is generally unchanged.
➤ First pass metabolism (the metabolism of a drug as it passes from the gut to the liver via the portal circulation before reaching the systemic circulation) is reduced due to reduced hepatic volume and blood flow.
➤ The volume of distribution of a drug depends on whether it is water-soluble or lipid-soluble. With age the ratio of fat–lean muscle increases; therefore lipid-soluble drugs such as benzodiazepines have an increased volume of distribution leading to prolonged effects and water-soluble drugs such as alcohol and digoxin have a smaller volume of distribution leading to more rapid peak effects.
➤ Serum albumen is reduced in chronic illness and malnourished patients and falls abruptly during acute illness whereas α-1-acid glycoprotein increases in acute illness. Acidic drugs like warfarin, aspirin, phenytoin and benzodiazepines bind albumen, whereas basic drugs like lignocaine and propranolol bind α-1-acid glycoprotein. Hence plasma protein binding of drugs can be altered in

acute illness and the free plasma concentration, which is responsible for drug effects, can be altered by the displacement of one bound drug for another. This mechanism is the basis of many drug interactions.

➤ Many drugs are cleared by the kidneys and renal drug clearance consistently declines with age. Renal blood flow falls by about 10% per decade of adult life, renal mass also declines and the number of nephrons decreases from 1 million to about 600,000 by age 80. Serum creatinine is not a good guide to renal function in older people and the Modification of Diet in Renal Disease (MDRD) formula is currently recommended for estimating glomerular filtration rate (GFR).[4]

➤ Hepatic blood flow and mass decline with age but in contrast to renal clearance, no reliable formula exists to estimate hepatic drug clearance. Cytochrome P450, esterases and alcohol dehydrogenases are enzymes of phase I metabolism and while enzyme activities are well maintained there is a quantitative reduction in phase I metabolism with age as a consequence of reduced mass and blood flow. Conjugation pathways responsible for phase II metabolism have been less well studied but seem to be well maintained in healthy older people but reduced in the frail.

ALTERATIONS TO PHARMACODYNAMICS WITH AGEING

➤ Pharmacodynamics refers to the effect of a drug on the body and for a given concentration of drug, older people often have an increased drug effect. This increased sensitivity is largely related to reduced haemostatic reserve in key organ systems; such as reduced β receptor numbers, reduced haemostatic reserve in the cardiovascular system, reduced baroreceptor responsiveness, impaired cognition, balance, thermoregulation and extrapyramidal function.

PHARMACOGENETICS

➤ Genetic polymorphisms of genes encoding drug metabolising enzymes increase risk of ADRs and therapeutic failure. Of the Caucasian population, 7–10% have a non-functional CYP2D6 (Cytochrome P450 family) gene resulting in reduced capacity to activate prodrugs like donepezil, rivastigmine, galantamine and tamoxifen. CYP2D6 polymorphisms are also implicated in ADRs with neuroleptics and antidepressants.

GENDER DIFFERENCES IN DRUG METABOLISM

➤ Liver mass is higher at all ages in males and declines in both sexes with age. Gastric motility is affected by sex hormones and is slower in women than men. Gastric alcohol dehydrogenase activity is reduced in women and this together with reduced volume of distribution contributes to higher alcohol levels in females after an equivalent drink.

FRAILTY, DISEASE AND DRUG METABOLISM

➤ Chronic frailty is associated with reduced activities of plasma esterases, decreased conjugation and drug clearance over and above those attributable to age alone. Further decrements in drug metabolism occur during acute illness, e.g. pneumonia, hip fracture, head injury, delirium.

BETTER PRESCRIBING IN OLDER PEOPLE

Understanding the effects of age and illness on drug metabolism is essential to guide good prescribing principles in older people, improve the quality of medical care for older people and reduce healthcare costs. There are a number of strategies that can be adopted to decrease the risk of potential problems.

➤ Avoid unnecessary prescribing and consider non-pharmacological treatment, if possible.
➤ Balance risks and benefits of a given agent.
➤ For prophylactic treatment consider comorbidities, risks of medication, likelihood of compliance and the population from which the evidence was identified.
➤ Review drugs regularly and withdraw unnecessary agents if possible.
➤ Start with a low treatment dose and increase slowly with close monitoring.
➤ Encourage patients to alert physicians, pharmacists and other healthcare professionals to symptoms that occur when new drugs are introduced.
➤ Physicians with a responsibility for older people in an institutional setting should develop a strategy for monitoring and reviewing their drug treatment.
➤ For those ADRs that come to clinical attention, it is important to review why they happened and to plan for future prevention.
➤ Report, via the appropriate postmarketing surveillance scheme, any ADRs encountered.
➤ Multidisciplinary education about the nature of physiological ageing and its effect on drug handling, and the possible presentations of drug-related disease in older patients.

Two strategies have recently been developed to identify older people at risk of adverse effects and reduce the risk of initiating drugs likely to cause adverse effects.
➤ STOPP (Screening Tool of Older Persons Prescriptions) comprises 65 clinically significant criteria for potentially inappropriate prescribing in older people.[5]
➤ START (Screening Tool to Alert doctors to Right Treatment) consists of 22 evidence-based prescribing indicators for commonly encountered diseases in older people.[5]

COMPLIANCE

Poor compliance with medication is an important problem in older people, occurring in between 40 and 75% of prescriptions and the consequences may be serious. Three common forms of drug treatment non-compliance are found in older people: overuse and abuse, forgetting, and alteration of schedules and doses.
➤ Some older patients who are acutely ill may take more than the prescribed dose of a medication in the mistaken belief that more of the drug will speed their recovery. Such overuse has clearly been associated with ADRs.
➤ Forgetting to take a medication is a common problem in older people and is especially likely when an older patient takes several drugs simultaneously. Data suggest that the use of three or more drugs a day places older people at particular risk of poor compliance. As many as 25% of older people take at least three drugs and older hospitalised patients typically take eight drugs simultaneously. Problems may also arise when dementia or depression is present, which may interfere with memory.
➤ The most common non-compliant behaviour of older people appears to be under-use of the prescribed drug. Inappropriate drug discontinuation may occur in up to 40% of prescriptions, mostly within the first year.
➤ As many as 10% of older people may take drugs prescribed for others and more than 20% may take drugs not currently prescribed by a physician.

Compliance with medication can be improved by careful explanation of the reasons for treatment, expected drug effects and side effects, use of medication lists, blister packs or dossett boxes and better labeling of medication. Recent studies in heart failure have shown that nurse specialists can improve compliance in older people and reduce mortality and morbidity.

Key points
- Whenever possible, alternatives to medication therapy should be considered as the initial treatment of choice in older people.
- Medications should be prescribed when indicated and not withheld due to a patient's age.
- Start with low doses and simplify dose and drug regimes.
- Keep the number of medications to the minimum possible to reduce the risk for adverse drug reactions and drug-to-drug interactions.
- Review medication regularly and especially prior to initiating new therapy
- Explain why the medication is needed and what effects and side-effects are to be expected.
- Follow-up care to review the efficacy and monitor any potential side effects is crucial.
- Timely discontinuation of a drug when therapeutic usefulness is surpassed is equally important.

REFERENCES

1 Royal College of Physicians. *Medication for Older People*. 2nd ed. London: Royal College of Physicians; 1997.
2 Fick DM, Cooper JW, Wade WE, Waller JL, Maclean JR, Beers MH. Medications to be avoided or used with caution in older patients. Updating the Beers criteria for potentially inappropriate medication use in older adults: results of a US consensus panel of experts. *Arch Intern Med*. 2003; **163**: 2716–24.
3 Department of Health. *National Service Framework for Older People. Medicines and Older People*. London: Department of Health; 2001.
4 Coresh J, Stevens LA. Kidney function estimating equations: where do we stand? *Curr Opin Nephrol Hypertens*. 2006; **15**: 276–84.
5 Gallagher P, Ryan C, Byrne S *et al*. STOPP (Screening Tool of Older Persons Prescriptions) and START (Screening Tool to Alert doctors to Right Treatment). Consensus validation. *Int J Clin Pharmacol Ther*. 2008; **46**: 72–83.

CHAPTER 7

Principles of rehabilitation

The emphasis in this chapter is on stroke survivors, lower-limb amputees, and patients with rheumatic and orthopaedic disorders.

Rehabilitation is defined by the WHO as an active process by which people who are disabled by injury or disease achieve a full recovery or realize their optimal physical, mental and social potential and are integrated into an appropriate environment.

DEFINITION OF IMPAIRMENT, DISABILITY AND HANDICAP

Impairment is loss or abnormality of psychological, physiological or anatomical structure or function.

Disability is a restriction or inability to perform a task or activity that is considered normal.

Handicap is social disadvantage suffered as a result of ill-health compared to a normal person of same age, sex and background.

Rehabilitation is a complex process and requires a skilled team with effective leadership. Success is usually measured in terms of the extent to which a person returns to a normal lifestyle. In many cases successful rehabilitation may mean some degree of acceptance of disability by the patient, and provision of some alternative means of achieving tasks that cannot be done independently. Rehabilitation is an important factor in old age medicine as:

➤ acute illness in older people often has functional consequences (especially mobility and self-care)
➤ many degenerative disease processes (osteoarthritis, ischaemic heart disease, peripheral vascular disease, chronic lung disease, stroke, osteoporosis) are age-related
➤ the prevalence of disability increases with age.

The principles of rehabilitation and the processes involved in older people are outlined in Tables 7.1 and 7.2.

TABLE 7.1 Key principles of rehabilitation in older people

Wholeness	Address the whole person rather than a part
Individualised	
Emphasis on functional abilities	Self-care, mobility, life spaces and leisure
Not time limited	Wider vision than hospital care
Active, planned responses	Requires a creative problem-solving approach

TABLE 7.2 The clinical process of rehabilitation

Key tasks	Processes used
Recognition of potential	Multidisciplinary team assessment
Rehabilitation goal setting	Multidisciplinary team meeting (with patient)
Re-ablement	General and special techniques
Regular Review	Further assessment
Resettlement	Home-visits, follow-up, liaison with primary care team
Readjustment	Empowering by education about disability and available services

Rehabilitation goals are highly focused statements of intent, generated from the assessment process and then agreed. Using goals has been shown to lead to improved outcomes provided that significant patient involvement occurs, and that both short- and long-term goals are developed. Goals need to be **S**pecific, **M**easurable, **A**chievable, **R**ealistic and **T**imed (SMART).

There are a number of systemic reviews for rehabilitation topics of relevance to older people, including falls, fractured neck of femur, stroke, etc. Most studies describe the effects of complex, multi-component interventions but in many cases the critical factor for successful rehabilitation remain undefined.

Comprehensive geriatric assessment (CGA) is a multidimensional interdisciplinary diagnostic process focused on determining an older person's medical, psychological and functional capability in order to develop a coordinated and integrated plan for treatment and long-term follow-up (*see* Table 7.3).

TABLE 7.3 Components of comprehensive geriatric assessment

Components	Elements
Medical assessment	Problem list Comorbid conditions and disease severity Medication review Nutritional status
Assessment of functioning	Basic activities of daily living Instrumental activities of daily living Activity/exercise status Gait and balance
Psychological assessment	Mental status (cognitive) testing Mood/depression testing
Social assessment	Informal support needs and assets Care resource eligibility/financial assessment
Environmental assessment	Home safety Transportation and tele-health

Frail older people benefit most from this type of assessment and it is recommended that it should be performed by a multidisciplinary team consisting of:
➤ A senior specialist physician in medical care of older people.
➤ A coordinating specialist nurse with experience in older people.
➤ A senior social worker, or a specialist nurse who is also a care manager with direct access to care services.
➤ Dedicated appropriate therapists.

Benefits of CGA include:

➤ Reduced short-term mortality.
➤ Increased chance of living at home.
➤ Improvement in physical function.
➤ Reduction in hospital readmissions and placement in care homes.
➤ Improved quality of life and cognition.

DISCHARGE PLANNING

➤ This is the development of a discharge plan for the patient prior to leaving hospital, with the aim of
 — improving patient outcomes
 — reducing length of stay and readmission rates
 — improving coordination of services following discharge bridging the gap between hospital and place of discharge
 — reducing inappropriate placement in nursing and care homes.
➤ To be effective, discharge planning should:
 — start as soon as possible after admission
 — involve a multidisciplinary team assessment covering medical, physical and functional activity, psychological assessment and social care needs
 — include an integrated package of care, covering both the hospital and community and tailored to the needs of the individual.

AIDS AND APPLIANCES:

A large range of aids for older people, mobility products and daily living aids are now available to help older patients maintain functional independence. These include mobility scooters, wheelchairs, walkers, frames, exercise equipment, orthopaedic supports, personal care products, bathing aids, footcare products and smaller items such as hand reachers, walking sticks, jar openers and pill boxes. Occupational therapists and physiotherapists can usually advise on and provide aids and appliances to facilitate mobility and independence.

As well as these physical aids, a number of agencies, such as CarelineUK, provide 24-hour *telecare monitoring services* for users in the event of a fall, emergency or crisis. This facility enables many older people to live a much more independent and active lifestyle, reduce need for nursing and residential care and reduce worry and anxiety for the client and their carers.

In addition to emergency alarms, there are sensors that monitor a range of variables including: temperature, movement, wandering (particularly useful for people with cognitive impairment), or data reporting leaks from gas-type devices, etc. When a sensor is activated it sends a signal to a central unit where trained advisors can take the most appropriate action, whether it's contacting a local key holder, doctor or the emergency services.

PREVENTION OF COMPLICATIONS (PRESSURE SORES AND CONTRACTURES)

Pressure ulcer prevention should be addressed at the earliest opportunity in older patients who are ill and immobile. Lying on a hard surface, such as a hospital trolley, for as little as 30 minutes can result in the development of a pressure ulcer which can cause considerable discomfort and disability, slow rehabilitation and delay discharge. Recommendations for prevention include:
➤ A formal pressure area risk assessment (e.g. Waterlow score) is recommended for all older patients.

➤ Pressure area skin inspection (sacrum and heels) on admission and at least daily in patients who remain immobile.
➤ Regular repositioning.
➤ Early mobilisation.
➤ All patients at high risk should be rested on high specification pressure-relieving mattresses and additional pressure-relieving heel protection where indicated.
➤ The finding of early or superficial skin damage should trigger appropriate care – which can prevent or reverse many impending ulcers.
➤ Risk factors such as pressure, shearing forces, friction, incontinence, pain and malnutrition should be addressed.
➤ Early referral to an expert on tissue viability if problems arise.

A contracture is defined as chronic loss of joint mobility as a result of structural changes in non-bony tissue, namely muscles, ligaments and tendons.
➤ It usually results from immobilisation due to injury or disease such as nerve injury, spinal cord damage, stroke or disease of muscles, tendons and ligaments.
➤ In addition to loss of joint motion contractures can cause significant pain thereby having significant functional consequences depending on the joint(s) involved.
➤ Prevention is achieved by a programme of positioning, appropriate splinting and range of motion exercises either manually or mechanically aided. For best results early intervention in immobilised patients is essential.
➤ Treatment involves joint mobilisation and stretching of soft tissues, mechanical techniques such as continuous passive motion machines, casting or splinting techniques, surgery and botulinum toxin injections for spasticity. The prognosis depends on the cause but in general earlier treatment produces best results.

STROKE REHABILITATION
➤ Stroke is a major health problem in the UK.
➤ Stroke care costs about 7 billion per year in the UK.
➤ It accounts for about 11% of all deaths and is a significant cause of morbidity.
➤ Approximately 110 000 people have a first or recurrent stroke each year.
➤ More than 900,000 people in England are living with the effects of stroke, with half of these being dependent on other people for help with everyday activities.

The National Stroke Strategy[1] outlines an ambition for the diagnosis, treatment and management of stroke, including all aspects of care from emergency response to life after stroke. The development of thrombolysis and other acute treatments has led to an increased emphasis on acute management of stroke but rehabilitation is still essential and must start from the beginning (see NICE, RCP and SIGN guidelines).

Evidence from clinical trials shows that patients managed in an organised *stroke unit* are more likely to survive, return home and regain independence that those who receive conventional care on a general ward. Current guidelines recommend that all patients with acute stroke should be admitted directly to a specialist acute stroke unit following initial assessment. After initial assessment and treatment the patient should be transferred to a specialist stroke rehabilitation unit or specialist stroke rehabilitation services in the community. A stroke unit is defined as:
➤ a discrete area in the hospital
➤ staffed by a specialist stroke multidisciplinary team
➤ access to equipment for monitoring and rehabilitating patients
➤ regular multidisciplinary meetings occur for goal setting
➤ provision of information and education for staff, patients and carers.

Rehabilitation is a cornerstone of modern acute stroke care. Although most therapy interventions have not been subjected to randomised controlled trial, they have been derived from extensive experience. Early mobilisation programmes aim to reduce secondary complications of immobility such as infection, venous thromboembolism, orthostatic hypotension and infection and to position patients in order to reduce the likelihood of contractures and shoulder subluxation, and avoid hypoxia.

Ongoing rehabilitation uses a wide variety of treatments and techniques to reduce activity limitation, often through improving motor control. There is much debate about the amount of therapy that is needed and whether there is a minimum threshold, below which there is no benefit at all. However, there is agreement that the treatment needs to be patient centered and incorporate a multidisciplinary process in which a number of disciplines carry out assessments and identify the range of problems. The multidisciplinary process involves a goal-planning cycle in which the patient is assessed, a problem identified, a recovery goal is set, an intervention is provided and then the process is reassessed. The setting of goals is central to effective and efficient rehabilitation. The process can occur on several time-scales and involve both short and long-term goals. Close cooperation and liaison is essential to ensure compatible goals and objectives. The first step is to achieve reasonable sitting balance, then move on to standing and transfers and then to walking. Reassessment is essential to identify progress and define any potential barriers to successful rehabilitation, which may be physical (e.g. pneumonia), psychological (e.g. depression), social (e.g. unsuitable housing), or cultural (e.g. patients and/or families reaction to disability).

The key members of the multidisciplinary team are:

➤ *Doctors* need to a have knowledge of the diagnosis, prognosis and complications of stroke. Both hospital doctors and GPs are essential in providing comprehensive and integrated acute and long-term care.

➤ *Nurses* play a central role, providing for the daily needs of patients, preventing complications, providing regular assessments of progress and support for patients and family.

➤ *Physiotherapists* are largely concerned with the recovery of movement and are involved in assessing motor and sensory function, advising and managing position and handling issues, training in walking and the provision of aids and preventing complications (especially respiratory).

➤ *Occupational therapists* play a key role in the recovery of functional tasks. They provide detailed assessments of activities of daily living and other aspects of occupational performance, including assessing visuo-spatial function, providing aids and appliances and assessing patients' abilities within the home setting.

➤ *Speech and language therapists.* Swallowing difficulties occur in a third of patients after stroke and it is vital that this is recognised early to reduce risk of complications. Often it recovers in a week or two and all that is required is careful feeding and thickened fluids. In more severe cases a nasogastric tube for feeding may be necessary and if the problem persists a feeding gastrostomy may be required. Impairment of speech is devastating to most patients. Speech therapists can help make the best use of whatever modalities of communication remain and advise family and staff about how best to communicate. Correction of other impairments such as deafness or reduced sight can often aid communication.

➤ *Clinical psychologists* are frequently involved in managing psychological and behavioural complications of stroke.

➤ *Social workers* help access services and facilities within a community setting.

➤ *Dieticians* advise on the management of nutritional problems and feeding regimens for enteral feeding.

➤ *Psychiatrists* advise on the management of affective complications of stroke.

➤ *Opthalmologists* help in the management of patients with visual problems.
➤ *The stroke coordinator* is often a senior nurse and helps coordinate all aspects of care from acute to community, facilitates the MDT working and has an important educational role for patients, cares and staff.

The outcome with rehabilitation is dependent on a number of factors including:
➤ Severity of initial deficit (*see* Table 7.4).
➤ Extreme frailty.
➤ Premorbid functional level.
➤ Haemorrhagic rather than ischaemic stroke.
➤ Prolonged drowsiness.
➤ Depression.
➤ Presence of intercurrent disease and other comorbidities such as cardiac failure.
➤ Location of the stroke: infarction of the non-dominant hemisphere may produce unilateral neglect, visuo-spatial and topographical disorientation which influence recovery and function, dysphasic patients with severely limited comprehension have particular problems, extensive cortical sensory loss is also regarded as a poor prognostic sign and more subtle defects that adversely affect outlook include intellectual impairment, apraxia, denial, impaired memory and motor perseveration.

TABLE 7.4 Markers of stroke severity

Unconscious during the first 24 hours
Incontinence of urine
Perceptual impairments
Loss of proprioception
Cognitive impairment

Recovery from stroke occurs over at least three months, and in some cases may continue for over a year. Little research has been done on later recovery but measurable recovery beyond a year is probably uncommon. The spontaneous recovery is due to resolution of cerebral oedema surrounding the damaged brain, and relearning of skills. Current guidelines recommend regular review to determine need for further rehabilitation after discharge.

LOWER LIMB AMPUTEE REHABILITATION
➤ The average age of people undergoing lower limb amputation is 70 and 25% are over 80 years of age.
➤ The majority have peripheral vascular disease.
➤ Comorbidities such as cardiovascular disease, cerebrovascular disease, chronic lung disease and diabetes are frequent.
➤ The loss of a limb in older people seriously threatens independence.
➤ Older amputees are a high-risk group with up to 50% dying within the next 3 years often as a result of cardiovascular or cerebrovascular disease.
➤ 25% of non-diabetics and 50% of diabetics require another amputation within the next 5 years.
➤ Studies have shown that older people are less likely to achieve community mobility than younger patients but the reasons for this are unclear. Nonetheless, with appropriate rehabilitation and social support the majority of older amputees can return home and lead functionally useful lives so this should always be offered and encouraged.

Rehabilitation after lower limb amputation typically involves three stages:

1 *Preoperative assessment*: The patient should be referred to a physiotherapist preoperatively, if possible. This allows time to improve strength and optimise mobility and functional status. It is also an opportunity to inform the patient and carers of the rehabilitation programme and expected outcome.

2 *Postoperative care*: Initial physical therapy is aimed at stabilising residual limb volume by decreasing oedema and promoting healing. The use of early walking aids improves functional recovery. A typical programme would include:
   — Days 1–3: bed exercises to strengthen arms abdominal muscles, lower back and remaining leg and balance training in the sitting position. A full range of hip and knee extension is required to maintain joint mobility and avoid contractures.
   — Days 4–6: training in transfers from bed to chair and wheelchair mobility is initiated. Balance and walking training with a walking frame is started.
   — Days 7–10: an early waking aid such as a pneumatic post-amputation aid is introduced, initially twice daily for 10 minutes increasing to 1 hour twice daily over 1–2 weeks.

3 *Prosthetic programme*: Patients should be referred to a specialist prosthetic centre for multidisciplinary assessment to decide on a functional or cosmetic prosthesis or recommend an alternative form of functional independence, for example a powered wheelchair. A prosthesis should be fitted if possible, as it facilitates transfers and standing and has cosmetic value. Limb fitting usually begins about 3 weeks postoperatively after below-knee amputation, provided wound healing is satisfactory. Prosthetic training focuses on stump care and bandaging, transferring and hopping with use of an aid. The programme then continues, where feasible, with improving balance and general fitness and walking on slopes and rough ground. Unfortunately, the energy expenditure required for mobilising with an above-knee amputation is beyond the capacity of many older patients, especially those with cardiorespiratory problems, and they are limited to wheelchair mobility.

Outcome of rehabilitation in lower limb amputation

➤ The functional outcome depends on a number of factors including:
   — the level of amputation
   — pre-morbid health (especially cardiovascular status)
   — comorbidities
   — psychosocial factors
   — patient motivation
   — stump pain, phantom sensations and phantom pain.

REHABILITATION IN RHEUMATIC AND ORTHOPAEDIC DISORDERS

Arthritis and other rheumatic disorders are among the most prevalent chronic health problems in older people, often leading to reduced functional activity, falls and loss of independence. Joint pain and arthritis causes difficulties with mobility, upper extremity function, household management and self-care activities. Effective management of arthritis in older people should include concurrent pharmacologic and non-pharmacologic interventions with targeted goals of pain relief, and preservation of functional independence and quality of life. The American College of Rheumatology (ACR) guidelines (2000) for the management of hip and knee arthritis highlight the importance of non-pharmacologic measures to relieve pain, and improve joint biomechanics and overall function (*see* Table 7.5).

TABLE 7.5 Management of osteoarthritis

Non-pharmacological	Pharmacological
To relieve pain Ice, heat, ultrasound, TENS	Analgesic medication Topical salicylate or capsaicin Adjunctive agents (tricyclic antidepressants)
To relive pain and improve joint mechanics Mobility aids (sticks, frame, etc.) Orthotic devices Weight reduction if obese	Arthrocentesis with intra-articular glucocorticoids or hyaluronic acid for knee arthritis
To improve muscle strength and conditioning Physical therapy Resistive exercise training Aerobic conditioning	
Pain still limiting function in spite of maximal therapy Chronic pain management if unsuitable for surgery	Surgical evaluation

Physiotherapists play an important role in management of the patient with arthritis and rheumatism and can:
➤ assess joint function and associated limitations
➤ advise on and supervise exercise programmes to improve joint biomechanics and mobility. Resistive training and aerobic exercises have been shown to improve physical performance, painful symptoms and reports of disability after 3 months
➤ use physical therapy such as ice, heat, ultrasound and TENS to relieve pain
➤ advise on aerobic exercise to assist weight loss.

Occupational therapists can:
➤ assess functional limitations
➤ provide therapy to maintain and or improve function
➤ advise on splints, aids, assistive devices and other adaptations to facilitate independence.

Podiatrists may also be involved and can:
➤ advise on orthotic devices and shock-absorbing shoes that have been shown to compensate for functional defects and are protective.

Dieticians provide:
➤ dietary advice to the obese patient, as weight reduction may significantly reduce pain by reducing biomechanical stress on weight-bearing joints.

REHABILITATION AFTER HIP FRACTURE (*SEE* CHAPTER 42 ON ORTHOGERIATRIC SERVICES)
➤ Hip fracture is common in older people with about 70 000 per year in the UK. The incidence is increasing and predicted to be 101 000 by 2020.
➤ The 1-year mortality rate after hip fracture is about 30%.
➤ A significant proportion of survivors fail to regain their previous functional level and need increasing care in the community or care home placement.
➤ Comorbidities are common.

The revised edition of the Blue Book, sponsored by the British Orthopaedic Association and the British Geriatrics Society, summarises current best practice in the care and secondary prevention of fragility fractures and sets six standards for hip fracture care. Together with the web-based National Hip Fracture Database, it allows trauma units to benchmark and improve their management of this serious and common osteoporotic injury. Rehabilitation needs to commence as soon as possible after surgery to promote independent mobility and function. A dedicated multidisciplinary team and involvement of orthogeriatricians is essential to assist medical management, rehabilitation and early discharge planning is important. The new guidelines place increasing emphasis on falls and bone health assessment as well as rehabilitation after injury.

➤ *Physiotherapy* should start on day of surgery if possible focusing on prevention of deep venous thrombosis, pressure sores, pneumonia and atelectasis, and constipation. The initial emphasis is on walking and activities of daily living (ADLs) such as transferring, toileting, washing and dressing. Balance and gait are essential components of mobility and useful predictors of functional independence. Decisions on weight bearing depend on the type of fixation, bone quality, fracture location and the patients' cognitive and functional ability to comply with graded degrees of weight bearing. In most patients, weight bearing with a standard walking frame is achieved in the first week after surgery. During week two, the patient can usually progress to crutches or sticks that allow faster walking and an improved gait pattern. Later the patient can progress to one stick held in the opposite hand. Many patients require extended rehabilitation either as inpatients or in the community (*see* Chapter 42 on orthogeriatric services). Exercise programmes to improve balance and coordination should be undertaken in the longer term to reduce risk of further falls.

➤ *Occupational therapists* work closely with the physiotherapist and play an important role in assessing and improving functional activities to facilitate independent living.

➤ *Dieticians* are essential as many older patients with fractured hips are malnourished and this can adversely affect the outcome of rehabilitation.

➤ *Social workers* play a vital role in facilitating discharge home with care or appropriate placement when this is required and must be involved early in the process.

Factors influencing the outcome of rehabilitation after fracture neck of femur include:

➤ pre-operative functional ability
➤ comorbidities
➤ cognitive impairment.

REFERENCE

1 Department of Health. *National Stroke Strategy*. London: Department of Health; 2007.

RECOMMENDED READING

American College of Rheumatology Subcommittee on Osteoarthritis Guidelines. Recommendations for the medical management of osteoarthrits of the hip and knee: 2000 update. *Arthritis Rheum*. 2000; **43**: 1905–15.

Cumming J, Barr S, Howe TE. Prosthetic rehabilitation for older dysvascular people following a unilateral transfemoral amputation. *Cochrane Database of Systematic Reviews*. 2009; **4**: art. no. CD005260.

Mulley GP. Principles of rehabilitation. *Rev Clin Gerontol*. 1994; **4**: 61–9.

National Institute for Health and Clinical Excellence. *Risk Assessment and Prevention of Pressure Ulcers. NICE clinical guideline 29*. London: NIHCE; 2001.

National Institute for Health and Clinical Excellence. *Pressure Ulcer Prevention: the use of pressure-relieving support surfaces (beds, mattresses and overlays) for the prevention of pressure ulcers in primary and secondary care. NICE clinical guideline 7.* London: NIHCE; October 2003.

National Institute for Health and Clinical Excellence. *The Management of Pressure Ulcers in Primary and Secondary Care. NICE clinical guideline 29.* London: NIHCE; 2005.

National Institute for Health and Clinical Excellence. *National Clinical Guideline for Diagnosis and Initial Management of Acute Stroke and Transient Ischaemic Attack (TIA). NICE clinical guideline 68.* London: NIHCE; 2008.

Royal College of Physicians of London. *National Clinical Guideline for Stroke.* 3rd ed. London: Royal College of Physicians; 2008.

Scottish Intercollegiate Guidelines Network. *Management of Patients with Stroke: rehabilitation, prevention, and management of complications and discharge planning: a national clinical guideline. SIGN guideline 64.* Edinburgh: SIGN; 2006.

Scottish Intercollegiate Guidelines Network. *Management of Hip Fracture in Older People. SIGN guideline 111.* Edinburgh: SIGN; 2009.

British Orthopaedic Association. *The Care of Patients with Fragility Fracture* (The Blue Book). London: British Orthopaedic Association; 2007. www.ccad.org.uk/nhfd.nsf/Blue_Book.pdf

CHAPTER 8

Domiciliary care for disabled older people

Given the high prevalence of chronic disease in older people, disability is a common problem. The majority of frail and disabled older people, including those with severe functional impairment, live in private households. Organising services for these patients requires careful assessment by a team approach to determine disease processes, functional ability, continence, cognition, mobility and social background. The National Health Service and Community Care Act (1990) (www.opsi.gov.uk/acts/acts1990/) gave local authority social service departments the lead responsibility for assessing individual need and planning, delivering and monitoring care for older and disabled people. The main objectives of the Act are:

➤ To promote domiciliary, day and respite services to enable older people to live in their own homes wherever possible.
➤ To provide practical support to carers, such as financial help and information about services.
➤ To assess need and have good management to ensure high-quality care.
➤ To promote the development of independent care providers.
➤ To clarify the responsibilities of care agencies; community care plans should show who is responsible for which services.
➤ To secure better value for taxpayers' money.

The characteristics and range of services provided by the different agencies are summarised in Table 8.1. In the past local authorities were the major providers of services for older people, but increasingly the independent sector plays a greater part in providing basic services like meals, home helps and respite care.

Informal carers, including family, friends and neighbours, provide a significant amount of the care. They are readily available and flexible and able to deal with unexpected events and emergencies. However, there is little recognised training or support for informal carers, many of whom are older and have their own health problems and they are often expected to do a job that few health professionals would consider feasible. It is important to recognise that informal carers need training to carry out many of the tasks of assisting disabled people. The best training is one-to-one with a therapist and carried out in the patient's home if possible.

Formal agencies have a larger pool of people and a range of technical expertise, skill and resources that may be essential for the patient, but are often less flexible and less available than informal carers.

TABLE 8.1 Summary of services provided for older patients in the community

	Services provided
Informal carers	Personal hygiene Domestic tasks Nursing tasks Financial help Counselling
Local authority social services	Home help Meals on wheels Social worker Respite care Occupational therapy Day centres Lunch clubs
Local health services	General practitioner District nurses Palliative care Macmillan nursing Pharmacist Podiatry Therapists (physiotherapy/speech and language) Dietician Continence advisory services Dental care Opticians Audiology services
Private services	Home care services Meals on wheels Respite care Nursing and residential homes Domiciliary nursing services Live-in companions
Voluntary services	National organisations (e.g. Age Concern, Help the Aged) Disease-or disability-specific organisations (e.g. Arthritis Council, Parkinson's Disease Society, Alzheimer's Disease Society) Organisations for carers (Crossroads www.crossroads.org.uk, Carers National Association www.carersuk.org) Locally oriented organisations (Citizens Advice Bureau, Women's Royal Voluntary Service) Culturally based services Lunch clubs Day centres Hospices Housing associations

EQUIPMENT

➤ A number of different aids and appliances are available that may help maintain functional ability, including:
  — hoists and transfer boards assist with lifting
  — walking sticks, crutches, frames and wheelchairs assist in maintaining mobility
  — battery-operated wheelchairs and tricycles are expensive, but help maintain outdoor mobility
  — stairlifts are expensive, but may be valuable for some patients.

➤ Given the individual nature of disability it is often difficult to determine what will suit a particular patient. A major difficulty in deciding what would be useful is the limited opportunity to test pieces of equipment, especially if they are expensive. Joint assessment by a physiotherapist and occupational therapist is the best way of ensuring the patient gets the right aids for both lifting and transfers and mobility.

SERVICES

➤ *Respite care* is used mainly to give carers a break from the burden of caring. It is a limited resource and, even when available, may be underused by carers who often find it difficult to accept their own needs for support and respite. Respite is usually provided in residential or nursing homes, depending on the physical and mental condition of the patient. Respite should be used as a valuable opportunity to reassess the patient and, where appropriate, provide treatment aimed at maintaining function.

➤ *Podiatry services*. Older patients often require the services of a podiatrist. Even simple problems like uncut nails and corns can render a patient housebound and immobile. The podiatrist can also treat congenital and acquired foot problems and recognise pedal manifestations of systemic disease such as vascular disease and peripheral neuropathy. Unfortunately, there are insufficient numbers of podiatrists to provide an adequate service to older people, many of whom are housebound and require domiciliary care.

➤ *Community psychiatric nurses* assess, treat and monitor all aspects of psychiatric illness, including dementia in older people, and liaise closely with consultant psychogeriatricians. They also have roles in education both with the patient and carer and support both, thereby playing an important role in maintaining mentally ill older people in the community.

➤ *Continence advisors* are experts in the management of both urinary and faecal incontinence and give specific advice on the continence aids available as well as their use by the patient and/or carer.

➤ *Dieticians*. Malnutrition is not infrequent in older people and is often unrecognised. Dieticians can assess and treat patients and provide valuable advice, especially in patients with swallowing difficulties who may have problems meeting their nutritional needs either orally or by enteral feeding.

➤ *Audiology services*. Hearing loss is common, affecting one in three older people, and can lead to withdrawal from society. Patients should be referred to an audiology clinic for assessment. The standard approach is to issue a hearing aid, but older patients often find these of little help or are unable to use them properly due to problems with manual dexterity, etc. Malfunctioning hearing aids are also a frequent problem and can usually be readily corrected by an ENT technician. Hearing therapists provide more comprehensive and continuous help, both practical and psychological, by trying to help the individual make the most of residual hearing, teaching them to use every available auditory and visual clues, and also how to use their hearing aid.

➤ *Meals on wheels* are usually administered by local authorities and are a means of providing one hot nutritious meal a day at low cost. Disadvantages include timing, provision, quality and ethnic requirements.

➤ *Luncheon clubs* provide inexpensive meals, act as social centres and are mainly used by active older people in the immediate neighbourhood.

➤ *Day centres* offer a wide range of activities, cater for a mixed client group and often provide transport for the less active.

➤ *The occupational therapist* (OT) role includes:
  — assessment of functional level
  — improving and maintaining function using graded tasks and activities to lessen fatigue and increase range of movements
  — restoring function by use of craft work, remedial games
  — assisting the permanently disabled to achieve maximum independence within the constraints of their disability
  — the use of activities to stimulate patients mentally and physically to maintain a sense of well-being
  — advising on appropriate aids and equipment.

➤ *Physiotherapists* work closely with the occupational therapists and help patients achieve maximum independence with minimal assistance. Their role involves:
  — assessment
  — providing therapy to improve, maintain and/or restore function
  — advising on appropriate aids and equipment.

➤ *Speech therapists* are involved in:
  — the assessment, treatment and management of communication disorders, including dysphasia, dysarthria, dysphonia, dyspraxia and dysfluency
  — the assessment, treatment and management of swallowing disorders
  — advising staff, relatives and carers about communication and swallowing.

➤ *Specialist teams* exist in some areas to provide an intensive level of support to selected clients following discharge from the acute sector or following a crisis. They are designed to gradually withdraw and let the usual services take over responsibility.

➤ *Social workers* work on behalf of the client in an advocacy role and enable them, through counselling, to cope with the problems of daily living and to obtain those services appropriate to their needs. They are responsible for:
  — assessment of the need for independent or social services residential or nursing home
  — reviewing financial ability to pay for care
  — housing adaptations
  — providing equipment for daily living
  — day care
  — day centres
  — respite care in residential and nursing homes.

ACTIVITIES OF DAILY LIVING (ADL)

These consist of the tasks undertaken daily to maintain personal care. Assessment includes ascertaining those activities that are deficient, evaluating the potential for improvement and deciding on a programme to achieve this potential.

➤ *Mobility*. All mobility must be considered and assessment of the environment (chairs, beds, stairs, toilet, etc.) is essential. Wheelchairs need skilled assessment to suit the needs of patients, carers and the environment.

➤ *Eating and drinking*. Special crockery and cutlery are available to assist the disabled person.

➤ *Toilet management.* This is an essential function for independence. Practical solutions such as handrails or a raised seat may be all that is required to maintain continence. Other solutions are commodes or chemical toilets, especially at night.

➤ *Personal hygiene and dressing.* Dressing practice and the use of aids may allow independence. Patients may require assistance, but should be encouraged to do as much as they can for themselves.

➤ *Communication.* Liaison with other members of the team ensures that patients with communication difficulties can receive therapy. Advice can be given on specific alarms and communication aids in the home.

➤ *Domestic tasks.* Training must be combined with knowledge of the patient's home circumstances and many patients perform better in their own homes than in the hospital environment. A visit to the patient's home enables assessment of the patient's ability to cope in the environment and what aids or adaptations may be necessary to facilitate this.

There are many instruments available to quantify activities of daily living (ADL), but the *Barthel Index* is the most popular and widely used in the UK. It is an ordinal scale and assesses levels of independence or dependence for 10 ADL tasks with a score of 0 (dependent) to 20 (independent).

The index is quick and easy to use and has been well validated. It can aid disability assessment and also show rehabilitation progress if repeated at intervals. The main disadvantage is that the steps on the scale are quite large and it is therefore not very sensitive to change. Also, especially for disabled people living at home, there is a marked ceiling effect in that patients can score a maximum of 20 points, but still have daily living restrictions. Extended ADL scales such as the *Nottingham ADL score* and the *Frenchay Activities Index* extend the range of the Barthel Index to include other important daily tasks such as housework, shopping and trips.

The Barthel Index
- Bowels
- Bladder
- Grooming
- Toilet
- Feeding
- Bed-to-chair transfers
- Walking
- Dressing
- Stairs
- Bathing

ASSESSMENT OF MENTAL FUNCTION

Given the high prevalence of dementia and cognitive impairment in older people, assessment of mental function is important. This usually involves a mental test score such as the Abbreviated Mental Test Score (AMTS) or the Mini-Mental State Examination (MMSE). The AMTS is a 10-point score and tests short- and long-term memory, orientation and numeracy skills. The MMSE is a 30-point score and tests orientation, short-term memory, concentration, language and comprehension. It is important to remember that these are screening tests and not diagnostic instruments. Deafness and speech impairments can make patients appear very cognitively impaired and depressed patients often score badly. Ethnic differences and level of education achieved may also affect scores. More complex tests are available to assess higher cognitive function and are usually applied by clinical psychologists.

Abbreviated Mental Test Score (AMTS)

- Age
- Time (to nearest hour)
- Address for recall
- Year
- Where do you live (town or road)?
- Recognition of two persons
- Date of birth
- Year of start of First World War
- Name of present monarch
- Count backwards 20 to 1

Mini-Mental State Examination (MMSE)

- Orientation in time (day, date, month, year, season)
- Orientation in place (place, level, street, city/town, country)
- Registration (three objects to repeat)
- Concentration (Serial sevens)
- Recall (the three objects above)
- Three-stage command
- Repeat 'no, ifs ands or buts'
- Read and obey command
- Write sentence
- Copy intersecting pentagons

CHAPTER 9

Legal aspects

LEGISLATION PROVIDING PROTECTION FOR OLDER PEOPLE WHO LACK CAPACITY
Mental Capacity Act 2005

The Mental Capacity Act 2005, which came into force in 2007, has brought changes into English law that clarify matters in respect of adults who lack capacity to make decisions.

The Act

- ➤ Clarifies the law dealing with the individual who lacks capacity.
- ➤ Codifies the law regarding 'capacity' and 'best interests'.
- ➤ Places advance decisions on statutory footing.
- ➤ Introduces the concept of substituted decision-making, lasting power of attorney (LPA) and independent mental capacity advocates (IMCA).

The Act is underpinned by five key principles:
- ➤ An adult is presumed to have capacity unless proven otherwise.
- ➤ Individuals should be supported as far as possible to make their own decisions.
- ➤ An unwise decision does not mean that an individual lacks capacity.
- ➤ A decision made for someone lacking capacity must be done in their best interests.
- ➤ Anything done for someone lacking capacity must be the option that least restricts their basic rights and freedoms.

Assessment of capacity

For the purposes of the Act, a person lacks capacity in relation to a matter if at the material time they are unable to make a decision for themselves because of an impairment or disturbance in the functioning of the mind or brain. This means that a person lacks capacity if:
- ➤ They have an impairment or disturbance that affects the way their mind or brain works; and
- ➤ The impairment or disturbance means that they are unable to make a specific decision at the time it needs to be made.

The question 'Is the person mentally incapable?' should be answered on the balance of probabilities (i.e. 'Is it more probable than not that the patient lacks the required mental capacity?'). In answering the question whether the person is unable to make the decision, one should seek to understand whether:

1 The person has a general understanding of the decision that they need to make and why they need to make it.
2 The person has a general understanding of the likely consequences of making or not making this decision.
3 The person is able to understand, retain and weigh up the information relevant to the decision.
4 The person can communicate their decision (by talking, using sign language or any other means).

Relevant information must include what the likely consequences of a decision would be and also the likely consequences of making no decision at all. In some cases it may be enough to give a broad explanation in simple language, while in others more detailed advice might be required. The more grave the consequences, the more important that the person understands the information relevant to the decision. Information should be presented in a way that is appropriate to meet the individual's needs and circumstances and it is important to use the most effective form of communication for that person.

Assessment of testamentary capacity
➤ A person is judged to have capacity to make a will if he or she:
  — knows the nature of action involved in making a will
  — has a reasonable grasp of the extent of their assets
  — knows the person or persons to whom they are leaving their property and money
  — is free of delusions, which might distort judgement.

Lasting power of attorney
➤ Lasting power of attorney (LPA) replaced the enduring power of attorney (EPA) on 1 October 2007 when the Mental Capacity Act came into force in England and Wales.
➤ EPA drawn up before 1 October 2007 can still be used and the donee should apply to register it with the Office of the Public Guardian. However, once the EPA has been registered it can not be revoked without the permission of the Court of Protection. The unregistered EPA can be revoked by signing a 'Deed of Revocation'.
➤ LPA can be drawn up at any time by a competent adult, but it has no legal standing until it has been registered with the Office of the Public Guardian.
➤ Unlike EPA or Power of Attorney, LPA can be drawn to give power to a trusted relative or friend to deal with financial, personal, social and health matters when an individual becomes mentally incompetent to make decision.
➤ LPA can also be set up to deal with property and financial matters only.
➤ Authority conferred by LPA is subject to any conditions or restrictions specified in the LPA and the provisions of the Mental Capacity Act 2005, and in particular to the principles of MCA and best interests.
➤ LPA can be cancelled at any time by an individual who has the capacity to do so. In case of dispute about whether LPA has been cancelled, the Court of Protection can be approached to make a decision.
➤ LPA does not authorise the donee to do an act that is intended to restrain a person unless three conditions are satisfied:
  — The patient must lack capacity in relation to the matter in question.
  — The donee must believe that the restraining act is necessary to prevent harm to the patient.

— The restraint must be a proportionate response to the likelihood of harm to the patient and the seriousness of the harm.

Curator bonis

➤ In Scotland courts could be asked to appoint a person as a curator bonis to manage affairs of person who had become mentally incapable of managing his/her affairs until 2002 when Guardians replaced them under the Adults with Incapacity (Scotland) Act 2002.

Best interests

➤ If no LPA has been appointed then decisions made must be in a person's best interests and the Mental Capacity Act 2005 helpfully provides a checklist to ensure that all relevant issues have been considered:
— determining best interests cannot be simply based on age, appearance, condition or behaviour
— all relevant circumstances should be considered
— every effort should be made to encourage and enable the person who lacks capacity to take part in the decision
— if there is a chance capacity will be regained, consider putting off the decision until this occurs
— particular caution must be applied to decisions about life sustaining treatment
— the person's past and present wishes and feelings, beliefs and values should be taken into account
— the views of others close to the individual should be considered.

Protection from liability

➤ Section 5 provides protection for actions carried out in connection with care (personal) or treatment including diagnostic and other procedures provided the action is carried out in the person's best interests and individual follows the Act's principles.

Advance decisions – *see* Chapter 10

The Court of Protection

➤ New court to deal with all areas of decision-making for incapacitated adults – this includes power to deal with matters concerning personal welfare or property and affairs including testamentary capacity.
➤ Court of Protection will have all the powers of High Court.
➤ Court may by order decide the matter or appoint a deputy to make decisions on behalf of an individual who lacks capacity.
➤ Court may decide whether a person lacks capacity to make a decision specified in the declaration.
➤ Court may decide on lawlessness of any act done, or yet to be done in relation to that person – this includes acts and omissions.
➤ Applications can be made by an individual member of family or through a solicitor.
➤ Examples of Court of Protection powers include:
— deciding where a patient lives
— deciding who (specified persons) can visit the patient
— making an order prohibiting a named person having contact with patient
— giving or refusing consent to treatment or continuation of treatment by a person providing healthcare for patient

— giving a direction that a person responsible for patient's healthcare allow a different doctor to take over this responsibility.

Court appointed deputy

➤ Powers of the deputy will be described and limited in scope and duration by the Court.
➤ The deputy may be requested where there is a risk of harm to an individual or where there is/are serious family dispute/s
➤ The deputy must be over 18 years of age and should not be a paid carer.
➤ In relation to property and financial affairs, a deputy may be directed to deal with cash, selling property or managing income.
➤ The deputy cannot refuse consent to life-sustaining treatment.
➤ The deputy cannot prohibit contact or ask another individual to take over healthcare responsibilities.
➤ The deputy is subject to limits on restraints (*see* Chapter 10).
➤ The Court can appoint more than one deputy.

IMCA (Independent Mental Capacity Advocate)

➤ An IMCA should be appointed if there are no suitable relatives or close friends ('unbefriended') to consult before decision is made in relation to:
— serious medical treatment
— NHS arranged accommodation or change in accommodation in hospital for 28 days or more or in care homes for 8 weeks
— local authority arranged accommodation for 8 weeks or more.
➤ Role of IMCA is to explore with the decision-maker the options to be considered, ascertain previous and present wishes of the patient and then advise on patient's best interests. He/she will have authority to examine medical records, talk to those involved in the patient's care and to talk to the patient.
➤ IMCA can challenge decision but in such case ultimately decision will be made by the Court of Protection

Ill-treatment and neglect

Mental Capacity Act introduces a new criminal offence of ill-treatment and neglect. A person found guilty may be liable to imprisonment for a term of up to 5 years.

Deprivation of liberty safeguards (*see Chapter 10*)

➤ These safeguards were added to the Mental Capacity Act and implemented on 1 April 2009 with aim of reducing the risk of deprivation of liberty. These recognise that there may be occasions when depriving a patient who lacks capacity of their liberty is necessary to protect them from harm and would be in their best interests.
➤ The guidance recommends that the patients who lack capacity and are at risk of being deprived liberty must be identified by the home or hospital and authorisation obtained from relevant local authority for those in care homes or Primary Care Trust, for those in hospital.

COMPULSORY ADMISSION AND TREATMENT OF PATIENTS WITH A PSYCHIATRIC ILLNESS
Mental Health Act 1983/Mental Health Act 2007
Introduction

➤ This Act can be used for patients with any formal mental illness, including delirium and dementia, although it is unusual to use the Act for such patients, as treatment can be given under common law in the patient's best interests.

➤ Treatment under the Act only applies to treatment of the mental illness itself and not to any coexisting physical illness, although it is possible to treat a physical illness that is the cause of a symptom of a mental illness.

➤ Although doctors have the power to recommend compulsory admission under the Act, the main right to make a formal application rests with the social worker or a relative.

➤ Informal patients have the right to refuse treatment except in case of an emergency. Those formally admitted under Sections 2 and 3 can be given treatment without their consent.

➤ Mental Health Act 2007 made changes to several areas of MHA 1983 and these are:

— broad definition of mental disorder from 'mental illness, arrested or incomplete development of mind, psychopathic disorder and any other disability of or disorder of mind' to 'any disorder or disability of mind'

— excludes people with learning disability

— replaces 'treatability test' with 'appropriate treatment is available' for the patient (this applies to detentions under Section 3)

— broader range of professionals are allowed to exercise certain functions of the Act – specifically, the approved social worker role is changed to approved mental health practitioner (AMPH) and other professionals, such as occupational therapists and psychologists, will be eligible to become approved AMHPs

— the responsible medical officer is replaced by a responsible physician

— professionals other than doctors, i.e. occupational therapists, psychologists and social workers, will be allowed to become approved clinicians

— independent mental health advocates for someone who is:
  • a community patient
  • subject to guardianship under MHA 1983 or
  • is liable to be detained under MCA 1983 (but not by virtue of Sections 4, 5(2) or (4), 135 or 136).

➤ An advocate will have the right to meet with patient in private and interview professionals involved in the patient's care, right to inspect records/notes.

➤ Help provided by the advocate may include obtaining information about MHA provisions, conditions or restrictions an individual is subject to and medical treatment prescribed or given to the patient.

— electro-convulsive therapy will not be given to an individual with capacity without his/her consent, except for emergencies

— Mental Health Review Tribunals: duty of hospital managers to refer cases to MHRT applies to community patients and those admitted under Section 2

— definition of medical treatment: medical treatment is referred to as treatment which has a purpose of alleviating, or preventing a worsening of, the disorder or one of more of the symptoms and manifestations

— penalty for offence of ill-treatment: maximum penalty for neglect or ill-treatment increases from 2–5 years

— nearest relative (can include civil partners).

➤ In addition, a revised code of practice to MHA 1983 came into force on 3 November 2008. This includes:

— respect for individual patient's wishes and feelings (present and past)

— respect for religious beliefs, culture and sexual orientation

— minimising restrictions of liberty

— patient involvement in planning, developing and delivery of treatment

— avoidance of unlawful discrimination

— addressing patient's well-being and safety as well as ensuring that resources are used effectively, efficiently and in an equitable way to meet the needs of the patient
— ensuring that views of carers and other interested parties are considered
— avoidance of unlawful public.

Provisions of the Act

SECTION 2

➤ Allows formal admission to hospital for assessment, observation and subsequent appropriate treatment.
➤ Requires support/recommendation of two registered medical practitioners although in case of urgent need an application can be made on recommendation of one doctor
➤ The application can be made by the patient's nearest relative or an approved mental health professional or a person given power to act on the patient's behalf.
➤ The assessment period is 28 days.
➤ The grounds for application:
— the patient is suffering from a mental disorder of a nature and degree that warrant detention for assessment (or assessment followed by treatment)
— the detention is in the interests of the patient him or herself (health and safety) or for the protection of other people.
➤ Patient may appeal to Mental Health Review Tribunal within 14 days of detention.

SECTION 3

➤ Section 3 allows admission for compulsory appropriate treatment of mental disorder or illness for 6 months.
➤ The application procedure is similar to that for sectioning under Section 2, except that under this section the nearest relative must be consulted when an applicant is an approved mental health professional.
➤ The grounds for application include:
— the detention in hospital is the most appropriate way of providing the care and medical treatment of which the patient stands in need
— treatment is necessary for the health and safety of the patient and others
— the treatment is likely to alleviate or prevent deterioration of the condition
— the person has a mental disorder of a nature or degree which makes it appropriate to receive treatment in hospital.
➤ As with Section 2, the patient may be discharged by the responsible medical officer, the hospital manager or a nearest relative – nearest relative must give 72 hours notice to hospital manager but the RMO can refuse this if he/she feels this would be dangerous to the patient or others. At this stage, the nearest relative can bring the case before a mental health review tribunal.

SECTION 4

➤ Admission as an emergency by reason of 'urgent necessity', i.e. nearest relatives cannot cope with the patient's behaviour.
➤ There must be an immediate significant risk to the patient or others.
➤ The approved mental health professional recommending emergency treatment should, if practicable, have known the patient before and have seen him in the previous 24 hours.
➤ The period of detention: maximum of 72 hours, but this can be converted to 28 days by seeking a second specialist opinion.
➤ During the first 72 hours the patient has no right of appeal.

SECTION 5

➤ Provides holding power for a doctor or a nurse for forcibly detaining informal patients for up to 6 hours.

➤ The consultant (or deputy) can enforce the detention for 72 hours.

➤ This applies to patients receiving inpatient treatment for a physical condition, but not to patients being treated in the outpatient clinic or day hospital.

➤ Under Section 5(2), the responsible clinician/medical practitioner responsible for treating a patient can make an application to detain the patient in hospital by writing a report to the managers. If the medical practitioner in charge of clinical care of a patient is likely to be absent, they can nominate another in their absence.

➤ Under Section 5(4) (nurse's holding power) a nurse can detain patients who are receiving treatment for mental disorder as an inpatient in a hospital if the nurse feels that it is necessary to do so for their safety or for the safety of others and it is not practicable to get a doctor to attend to the patient for the purposes of preparing the report for application.

SECTION 7: GUARDIANSHIP

➤ This section allows the local authority (or a relative accepted by the local authority) to act as guardian to a person with a mental disorder and therefore provide community care.

➤ It may be used where there is conflict between the wishes of the relative and what is considered to be in the best interests of the patient.

➤ The guardian has power:
— to require an individual to live in a particular place but cannot restrict movement
— to require access to be given to doctors, social workers and others at any place where the individual lives
— to attend a particular place for treatment.

➤ Signatures of two registered medical practitioners (one of whom should be a specialist) are required by this section.

➤ The maximum duration is 6 months, but it is renewable for a further 6 months, then year to year.

SECTION 117

➤ This section applies to people detained under Sections 3 and 37 of the Mental Health Act 1983. Under this, the local authority, as well as the health authority, has a statutory duty to carry out joint assessment and provide services free of charge.

SECTION 135 AND 136

➤ These sections can be used to remove a person who is suffering from mental disorder to a place of safety.

Restraint of older patients (see Chapter 10)

➤ Freedom of movement is an important basic right enforceable through a writ of *babedes corpus*. The clinical use of restraint raises moral and ethical dilemmas, particularly when the individuals are too confused and, therefore, not competent to make a decision for themselves.

➤ While it is usually morally unjustifiable to restrain an older patient, there may be a case for using restraints in the case of patients who, because of their mental condition, are at risk of harming themselves. Under these circumstances, the law permits such an action as long as it is being performed in the best interests of the patient.

➤ Under Section 5(4) of the Mental Health Act a nurse is allowed to use the minimum force necessary to prevent a patient from leaving the hospital.

OLDER PATIENTS WHO DO NOT HAVE ACUTE PSYCHIATRIC ILLNESS BUT WHO ARE CONSIDERED TO BE AT RISK IN THEIR HOMES
National Assistance Act 1948 – Section 47

➤ The main function of this section is to remove an individual considered to be at severe risk at home, e.g. an older person with a fractured humerus who cannot look after themselves, but who refuses to go to hospital.

Grounds for use

➤ A person who is suffering from a grave and chronic disease or, being aged, infirm or physically incapacitated, is living in unsanitary conditions.
➤ A person who is unable to look after him/herself and is not receiving proper care and attention from others.

Requirement

➤ An order from a magistrate.
➤ Application usually made by a social worker on behalf of the local authority and supported by a community physician.

Patient and relatives

➤ Patient has a limited right of appeal and relatives have no say.

LEGISLATION GOVERNING PROVISION OF CARE AND SERVICES FOR OLDER PEOPLE
National Assistance Act 1948 – Section 21

➤ This Act empowers local authorities to provide accommodation for adults over 18 years of age who are:
— disabled
— ill
— in need of care as a result.
➤ In 1991 the Act converted power to duty to provide temporary accommodation to:
— those who have no alternative accommodation
— those who have urgent need because they have a mental disorder or to prevent mental disorder.

National Assistance Act 1948 – Section 29

➤ Under this section local authorities are empowered to:
— provide a social work service
— make arrangements for promoting the welfare of disabled persons (i.e. those who are deaf, blind, dumb or suffer from a mental disorder of any description or are handicapped as a result of illness, injury or other disabilities).

Chronically Sick and Disabled Persons Act 1970 – Section 2

➤ The section covers services such as practical assistance in the home, home adaptations, transport for a person to use services, meals and telephones.

Health Services and Public Health Act 1968 – Section 45

➤ Under this Act, social services are empowered to provide services to older people to promote their welfare, e.g. meals, home helps, day centres, home adaptations and social work support.

The National Health Service and Community Care Act 1990

➤ Under Section 47 of this Act the local authorities have the responsibility for planning, financing, delivery and regulation of community care services to vulnerable groups, including the old and mentally ill.

➤ In most areas local social services and health services have an agreed multi-agency body that acts as an eligibility panel for persons aged 65 and over and this panel considers the community care assessment and makes a decision as to whether an individual needs:
   — NHS continuing care provision for frail older people/mental health care of older people
   — nursing home placement
   — residential care placement
   — extra care sheltered accommodation
   — domiciliary/day-care packages of care requiring more than a notional maximum sum set by the local authority.

➤ Criteria for each of the above provisions are drawn up by the local authority after full consultation with health service providers. The cost of care is means-tested in England – those with assets of more than £22 500 have to pay the full cost of care home place while Council will pay for part of the costs of accommodation and personal care for those with capital of between £13 500 and £22 250 and pay full for those with capital of less than £14 000.

➤ In Scotland the personal care is free. Some councils assess care at person's home on income rather than value of individual's assets – the income must total less than the level of income support, plus 25%.
   In terms of contribution towards NHS-funded nursing care:
   — England introduced a new single band of £101 on 1 October 2007.
   — Scotland has a flat contribution of £149 per week for personal care, plus £67 per week for those assessed as needing nursing care.
   — Wales has a flat rate contribution of £114.90 per week towards nursing care.

The Carers (Recognition and Services) Act 1995

➤ This Act, which does not apply to Northern Ireland, enables local authorities to assess the needs of carers and individuals in need of community care services.

Caring about Carers – 1999

➤ Published by the government to stimulate diversity and flexibility in provision of breaks for carers or direct services to carers, in order to allow respite from the direct responsibility of supervising or caring.

The Social Work (Scotland) Act 1968

➤ Under this Act, social work departments are obliged to provide guidance, advice and assistance to people in need of care because of age, infirmity or because they have a physical illness or mental disorder.

Community Care (Delayed Discharges, etc.) Act 2003

➤ This Act has been introduced to help achieve a sustained reduction in the number of patients who are delayed in hospital, which will also free up NHS hospital beds for other patients.
➤ The Act aims to:
   — improve and strengthen discharge planning
   — improve timely provision of the services patients need to transfer from one care setting to another
   — strengthen local partnership working between the health services and the SSD.
➤ The Act addresses:
   — communication requirements between the hospital and the SSD
   — penalties for the SSD if a delay in the patient discharge is caused by the unavailability of services.

RIGHTS OF INSTITUTIONALISED OLDER PEOPLE

➤ All older people in an institution are by entry criteria disabled, and any assessment and treatment provided must take into account their needs, their dignity and autonomy.
➤ The National Standards Commission in line with Section 23 of the Care Standards Act 2000 (CSA) has set up standards, the aims of which are to provide measurable quality of life for older people using the services of the home (see below). Until 31 March, these regulations were carried out by the Commission for Social Care Inspection. The Health and Social Care Act 2008 established the Care Quality Commission, which took over the functions of Commission for Social Care Inspection as well as functions of Healthcare Commission and the Mental Health Act Commission, which had the monitoring function with regard to the operation of the Mental Health Act 1983.

STANDARDS APPLIED TO INSTITUTIONS PROVIDING CARE TO OLDER PEOPLE
Choice of home

➤ For an individual to make a decision they must have full information about the home. The Commission therefore requires the home to produce a statement of purpose, setting out its aims and objectives, the range of facilities and services it offers, and terms and conditions. In addition it is required that:
   — no older person should be admitted to a home without a full needs assessment
   — the services offered by the home should be able to meet the needs identified
   — an individual and their carers/relatives should be given the opportunity to visit and assess the services offered by the home.

Health and personal care
Privacy and dignity

➤ The home's philosophy of care must ensure that residents are treated with respect and dignity and their right to privacy is respected. This should cover dying and death.

Healthcare

➤ The home should not only promote and maintain health, but ensure access to healthcare services to meet the needs identified.

Medication
➤ While promoting self-administration in those who are able and willing to take on this responsibility, policy and procedures should follow guidelines laid down by the Medicines Act 1968, the Royal Pharmaceutical Society (RPS), the Misuse of Drugs Act 1971 and the United Kingdom Care Commission (UKCC).

Social contact and activities
➤ The routines of daily living and activities made available should be flexible and varied to suit and meet the expectations, preferences and capabilities of the individual, taking into account their social, religious and recreational interests.

Autonomy and choice
➤ Individuals should be helped to exercise choice and control over their lives and this covers meals and mealtimes.

Complaints and protection
➤ The home should ensure that there is a clear and accessible complaints procedure for use by individual residents and their relatives.
➤ The individual's legal rights should be protected.
➤ Protection from abuse/neglect – robust procedures should be in place to respond to any suspicion or evidence of abuse or neglect.

Environment
➤ The environment, including communal facilities, should be safe and well-maintained.
➤ Sufficient and suitable lavatories and washing facilities.
➤ Availability of specialist equipment to maximise independence, e.g. hoists, grab rails.
➤ Individual rooms should meet the needs of that person, e.g. a person in a wheelchair should have at least 12 square metres of usable space.
➤ Rooms should be furnished and equipped to assure comfort and privacy, and should meet the assessed needs of the individual. Where possible individuals should be allowed to bring in their own possessions.

Services
➤ All services (heating, lighting, ventilation) should meet the relevant environmental health and safety requirements and the needs of the individual.
➤ The home should be clean, pleasant and hygienic.

Staffing
➤ The skill mix of qualified/unqualified staff should be appropriate to the assessed needs of the residents.
➤ A minimum ratio requirement of 50% trained members of staff (NVQ Level 2 or equivalent) – recommended in 2005.
➤ Staff training and development programme should meet National Training Organisation (NTO) workforce training targets and ensures that staff fulfil the aims of the home and meet the changing needs of the residents.

Day-to-day operations
➤ The person in charge must be fit to be in charge, of good character and able to discharge their responsibilities fully, that is:
   — qualified, competent and experienced to run a home

— have at least 2 years' experience in a senior management capacity

— he/she should have a qualification, at Level 4 NVQ

— where nursing care is provided by the home, there should be a first-level registered nurse who has a relevant management qualification.

FURTHER READING AND INFORMATION

Department of Health. Information on Code of Practice for Mental Health Act 1983, www.dh.gov.uk/en/Healthcare/NationalServiceFrameworks/Mentalhealth/DH_4132161

Department of Health. *Mental Capacity Act 2005.* Department of Health; 2005. www.opsi.gov.uk/acts/acts2005/ukpga_20050009_en_1

Department of Health. *Mental Capacity Act 2005: code of practice.* London: The Stationery Office on behalf of the Department of Constitutional Affairs, Crown copyright; 2007. www.justice.gov.uk/guidance/mca-code-of-practice.htm

Department of Health. *Mental Health Act 2007.* Department of Health; 2007. www.opsi.gov.uk/acts/acts2007/ukpga_20070012_en_1

Department of Health. *Mental Capacity Act 2005: deprivation of liberty safeguards.* Consultation Paper CP23/07. Department of Health; 2007.

Department of Health. *National Minimum Standards and the Care Homes Regulations 2001.* 3rd ed. London: The Stationary Office; 2006.

For information on making and registering a LPA: www.publicguardian.gov.uk

ACKNOWLEDGEMENT

It is acknowledged that some of the information in this chapter comes from the Mental Capacity Act (2005) Code of Practice, issued by the Lord Chancellor on 23 April 2007 in accordance with Sections 42 and 43 of the Mental Capacity Act 2005 and published by the Department for Constitutional Affairs, London TSO (The Stationery Office).

CHAPTER 10

Ethical issues

1 PRINCIPLES OF MEDICAL ETHICS

Four widely accepted general principles of medical ethics employed in medical decision-making are:

1 *Autonomy* – respecting patients' wishes and facilitating and encouraging their input into the medical decision-making process.
2 *Justice* – an impartial and fair approach to treatment and the distribution of resources without discrimination on the grounds of age, race, sex, religion or sexual orientation.
3 *Beneficence* – to do good.
4 *Non-maleficence* – to do no harm.

2 CONSENT

2.1 The General Medical Council proclaims that:

➤ 'Patients must be able to trust doctors with their lives and well-being . . .' In particular as a doctor you must:
  — treat every patient politely and considerately
  — be honest and open and act with integrity
  — must make the care of patient his/her first concern
  — listen to patients and respect their views
  — give patients information in a way they can understand
  — respect patients' right to reach decisions about their treatment and care
  — make sure that your personal beliefs do not prejudice your patients' care.

2.2 The form of consent

➤ For a surgical procedure – written documentation or structured conversation is necessary.
➤ For a trivial intervention– patient's verbal agreement may be assumed to imply consent.

2.3 The law

The following outline summarises the principal elements of English consent law.

➤ Adults have a legal right to choose whether to consent to medical treatment, to refuse it or to choose one rather than another of the treatments on offer.
➤ Valid consent to medical intervention provides legal defence to the health worker from civil actions in battery (unconsented touching) or negligence, and from prosecution for the crime of battery.
➤ For actions in battery to succeed, the plaintiff must only prove that intentional touching occurred without consent; harm need not have occurred.

> ➤ The components of a legally valid consent are broadly that the person has capacity, has been informed about the intervention and provides the consent voluntarily.
> ➤ Adults are presumed legally competent until proven otherwise.
> ➤ The legal test of competence to consent is that the individual can comprehend and retain the relevant information, believe it, weigh the information by balancing risks and benefits, and finally arrive at a choice (which need not be a rational one).
> ➤ To avoid action in battery, a health worker need only provide information relating to the nature and purpose of the health intervention.
> ➤ To avoid action in negligence, a health worker must disclose that level of information considered to be proper by a responsible body of medical opinion.
> ➤ No adult can provide a legally effective consent (or refusal) to healthcare interventions being carried out on another adult.
> ➤ Where no consent is available because the patient lacks capacity and the patient has not made an advance decision or an LPA (lasting power of attorney), a health worker may legally treat the patient, so long as they act in the best interests of the patient or on the basis that the treatment is immediately necessary.

3 MENTAL INCAPACITY (*SEE* CHAPTER 9)

> ➤ The right of a mentally competent adult to refuse medical or any other intervention is enshrined in UK common law and reinforced by the Human Rights Act 1998 which incorporates the European Convention on Human Rights into domestic law.
> ➤ A person may refuse treatment for reasons that are 'rational, irrational or for no reason' and a doctor may be liable in assault or battery or for breach of Article 8 of the Convention on Human Rights if he or she touches a person contrary to his or her wishes.
> ➤ If the person is mentally incapable, whether temporarily or permanently, the doctor must act in line with the Mental Capacity Act 2005 and determine if the individual has made an advance decision or appointed an individual to make decision on his/her behalf using the lasting power of attorney (LPA). For LPA to be effective, it must be registered with the Office of the Public Guardian.
> ➤ If no LPA has been appointed and there is no advance decision then a decision must be made in the person's best interests.
> ➤ The Court of Protection can be asked to appoint a deputy if there is no LPA to make decisions – he/she may be authorised by the Court to make decisions on social and health matters but the deputy will not have the authority to refuse consent to life-sustaining treatment.
> ➤ A decision on mental capacity is ultimately a question of law for a court to decide. However, most decisions about mental capacity to make decisions about medical treatment never reach the hands of lawyers and are undertaken by the treating doctor
> ➤ Mental incapacity is a significant issue for doctors who provide healthcare for older people because of the high prevalence of both dementia and delirium.

3.1 Legal rules for assessing mental capacity for medical decisions

The Mental Capacity Act 2005[1] sets out a clear test for assessing capacity. The assessment is both decision and time specific and is based on the common law judgments set out in *Re C* (1994)[2] – a case in which the High Court was asked to decide whether a schizophrenic patient from Broadmoor Hospital was mentally competent to refuse amputation of a gangrenous leg, and the Court of Appeal case *Re MB* (1997),[3] concerning a pregnant woman.

In assessing capacity two questions need to be asked:
➤ Does the person have an impairment of the mind or brain, or is there some sort of disturbance affecting the way their mind or brain works? (It does not matter whether the impairment or disturbance is temporary or permanent.)

If so, does that impairment or disturbance mean that the person is unable to make the decision in question at the time it needs to be made?

The assessment is specific to the decision being undertaken and a person with borderline capacity may be able to make simple decisions concerning treatment of a straightforward nature, but unable to make a decision on a more complex issue.

The question 'Is the person mentally incapable?' should be answered on the balance of probabilities (i.e. 'Is it more probable than not that the patient lacks the required mental capacity?').

Everyone is presumed to be mentally capable until proved otherwise. However, once it is proved that a person is mentally incapable there is a presumption that this continues until the contrary is established.

In answering the question whether the person is unable to make the decision, one should seek to understand whether:

1   the person has a general understanding of the decision that they need to make and why they need to make it
2   the person has a general understanding of the likely consequences of making or not making this decision
3   the person is able to understand, retain and weigh up the information relevant to the decision
4   the person can communicate their decision (by talking, using sign language or any other means).

Relevant information must include what the likely consequences of a decision would be and also the likely consequences or making no decision at all. In some cases it may be enough to give a broad explanation in simple language while in others more detailed advice might be required. The more grave the consequences, the more important that the person understands the information relevant to the decision.

Information should be presented in a way that is appropriate to meet the individual's needs and circumstances and it is important to use the most effective form of communication for that person.

Section 3(3) of the Act sets out that people who can retain information for a short while must not automatically be assumed to lack capacity and that it depends on what is required for the particular decision in question. Items such as notebooks, photos, posters or recordings can help people to retain information.

The decision about mental capacity will vary according to the gravity of the decision – the more serious the decision, the greater the capacity required.

3.2 Mental capacity and the Mental Health Acts

Mental capacity is not relevant to the working of the Mental Health Act 1983 or Mental Health Act 2007 in England and Wales and the Mental Health (Scotland) Act 1984. The various sections of these Acts are not framed in terms of mental incapacity, but in terms of mental illness and the interests of the patient's health and safety and the protection of others. If applicable, the Acts allow the treatment of mental illness without the consent of the person. Although it is not possible to treat coexisting physical illness, it is possible to treat physical illness that is a cause or consequence of the mental illness. So it is possible to force-feed a patient with anorexia under the Act, whereas it is not possible to amputate a gangrenous leg simply because the patient has schizophrenia.

3.3 Mental capacity for non-medical decisions

The law relating to non-medical decisions and mental incapacity is generally similar to that for medical decisions. Presently, in England and Wales, there are a variety of slightly different common-law tests for determining mental capacity relating to different decisions, i.e. there is a specific test for mental capacity to make a will, to enter into a contract, to marry, etc. The Mental Capacity Act 2005 provides one uniform test for mental capacity and a single system of law governing the way in which decisions should be made for a mentally incapable adult, whether they be related to health, social welfare or finance.

4 CONFIDENTIALITY

➤ Confidentiality is one of the basic premises of medical practice.
➤ It is fundamental to a doctor–patient relationship based on trust.
➤ The GMC's *Duties of a Doctor*[4] states that doctors have a duty to respect the privacy of patients and to effectively protect the information given to them. This encompasses all information obtained in a professional capacity.
➤ The Human Rights Act 1998 also prevents health professionals from disclosing information given to them in confidence under Article 10 – the right to freedom of expression. If information is to be shared with others, then a patient's consent should always be obtained unless there are exceptional circumstances.
➤ But doctors have a duty of care not only to individuals but also to the rest of the community. The nature of information shared between doctors and their patients, and changes in medical practice can lead to conflicts of interest. When these occur and the question of breaching confidentiality arises, there must be clear ethical justification for doing so.

4.1 Sharing information with the patient's consent

➤ Consent must be obtained before disclosing information to another party, unless exceptional circumstances dictate otherwise. It is good practice to document this consent.
➤ Depending on the nature of the disclosure, this can be done formally with the patient's written consent or as a record that verbal consent has been given.
➤ To give consent the patient should understand the nature and effects of the disclosure and have the capacity to make the decision.
➤ Sharing information between health professionals to provide good healthcare is essential for good practice and therefore it is not always necessary to get explicit consent for this, provided that the patient has agreed to treatment or investigation. For instance, if a patient agrees to a specialist referral from their GP, then it is implied that they are happy for the GP to pass on details to the specialist. The specialist will, of course, receive the information in confidence.
➤ Sharing information within the healthcare team, including administrative and other staff, may be necessary in case of patients who are diagnosed with a serious communicable disease. In these situations it is necessary to obtain their consent.

4.2 Sharing information without consent

➤ This can occur in an emergency situation where it is impractical to obtain consent, or when patients decide to withhold consent or do not have the capacity to give it.
➤ The GMC offers guidance on situations when doctors may be justified in disclosing information that has been imparted to them in confidence, or when they are required to do so. These can be summarised as:

— when it is in the best interests of the patient

— when it is in the public interest, i.e when failure to disclose will put healthcare workers or other patients at risk, e.g. serious communicable disease

— when a known sexual contact of a patient with a sexually transmitted serious communicable disease are at risk

— when required to by statute or law

— approved under Section 251 of the NHS Act 2006 in England and Wales

— for the purposes of medical research and education, or public health.

➤ In cases where it has not been possible to obtain consent the patient should be informed of the decision to disclose information at the earliest opportunity. Breaching confidentiality, even when justifiable, remains an infringement of patients' rights and doctors should be prepared to defend these decisions. It may be advisable to discuss the matter with a colleague or a professional body before arriving at such a decision. Also it is advisable that doctors discuss this with the Caldicott Guardian and document it in the patient's records.

4.3 Legal and statutory processes

➤ In a court of law a judge can order the disclosure of information.

➤ A doctor can object if they believe the information to be irrelevant, but this decision ultimately falls to the judge.

➤ When lawyers or the police seek information this cannot be given without consent. The exception to this is where failure to do so would put people at risk of serious harm.

➤ Information must be disclosed where there is a statutory obligation to do so, for example in the notification of certain infectious diseases or in substance misuse.

➤ In counterbalance the Data Protection Act 1998 and the Human Rights Act 1998 (the right to freedom) confirm a responsibility to prevent disclosure of information that has been imparted in confidence particularly if doctors believe that disclosure is likely to cause serious harm to a person's physical or mental health.

4.4 Medical research, education and public health

➤ In broad terms, when information is to be used for research (audit, epidemiology), education and public health:

— information should only be given to those who are also bound by a duty of confidentiality

— consent should be sought to share information

— data should be anonymous if this will suffice.

4.5 Access to medical records

➤ Patients have a right to view their own medical records if they wish.

➤ Under the Data Protection Act 1998 a patient can expect to view or be supplied with a copy of their medical records.

➤ Information can be withheld if a doctor feels that it may be harmful to the patient or would compromise the confidentiality of others.

➤ In most cases the application for access to medical records is made in relation to insurance claims or employment. Information should only be imparted with the patient's written consent.

➤ Under the Access to Medical Reports Act 1988, the patient has a right to inspect or be supplied with a copy of their medical reports. However, reports prepared by an independent practitioner who has not treated the person and who has not been involved in his/her care is not covered by the Medical Reports Act or the Data Protection Act 1998.

5 ADVANCE DECISION/ADVANCE DECISION TO REFUSE TREATMENT

An advance decision (AD)/advance decision to refuse treatment (ADRT), otherwise known as an advance directive or a living will, is a statement of treatment preferences so as to indicate a person's wishes should the capacity for decision-making be lost in the future. Based on the principle of autonomy, it aims to project this forward into possible future mental incapacity.

➤ A professional must follow a verbal advance decision to refuse treatment if he/she consider that it exists and is valid and applicable except if treatment is life-sustaining.

➤ Prior to October 207 when Mental Capacity Act 2005 came into force, AD/ADRT were legally valid under common law.

➤ Article 5 of the Mental Capacity Act 2005 sets out the conditions that must be met for AD/ADRT to be legally valid. These are:
 — an individual making or drawing up advance refusal must be an adult aged 18 or over
 — the person must be competent or deemed to have capacity at the time the AD/ADRT is formulated
 — the AD/ADRT must specify the treatment that he/she wishes to refuse in medical and lay terms
 — the person can specify the circumstances in which the refusal will apply
 — the person making the AD/ADRT has not acted inconsistently with the terms of the refusal.

➤ AD/ADRT must be valid and applicable – it is not valid if it is subsequently withdrawn by the person or by the LPA (lasting power of attorney), appointed by the person. It is not applicable if the person has the capacity to make a decision at the time of treatment or the treatment has not been specified or unanticipated circumstances arise that are likely to have influenced the decision.

➤ AD/ADRT dealing with life-sustaining treatment must be written, signed and witnessed and include a statement that the decision applies even if the person's life is at risk.

➤ Refusal of non life-sustaining treatment can be verbal.

➤ The Mental Capacity Act 2005 applies to England and Wales. In Scotland, this area is covered by the Code of Practice issued under the Adults with Incapacity (Scotland) Act. In Northern Ireland, common law applies as there is no statute.

➤ Basic/essential care, which includes provision of food and water by mouth, warmth, shelter and basic nursing care to keep person comfortable or to reduce distress, such as use of analgesics, cannot be included in an advance statement by an individual.

6 ISSUES SURROUNDING PATIENTS' LIBERTY TO DRIVE AND THE LAW

➤ In the UK, the 1988 Road Traffic Act and the more recent Motor Vehicles (Driver Licences) Regulations 1996 define severe mental disorders as a relevant disability for licensing and this includes dementia.

➤ The person is obliged by law to inform the DVLA (Driver and Vehicle Licensing Authority) about their condition. If a patient refuses to do so despite advice from their doctor and family then the doctor can inform the DVLA after informing the patient of this decision.

➤ Professional codes of conduct usually allow for breaking of medical confidentiality in the case of considered assessments of dangerous driving when such drivers will not cease driving.

➤ Courts in the UK have considered that doctors are bound to advise patients on conditions which may impair safe driving.

7 CARDIOPULMONARY RESUSCITATION (CPR) AND DO-NOT-ATTEMPT-RESUSCITATION ORDER (DNAR)

➤ While CPR decisions are commonly made by hospital physicians, GPs may be involved in making such decisions if they are in charge of clinical care of patients in community hospitals.

➤ The new updated guidelines issued by professional bodies (British Medical Association [BMA], Royal College of Nursing and Resuscitation Council [UK])[5] incorporate several important changes, some of which have been included in recognition of the provisions of the Human Rights Act 1998, the Mental Capacity Act 2005 (England and Wales) and the Adult with Incapacity (Scotland) Act 2000.

➤ When making the DNAR decision it is important to recognise that:
  — The goal of medicine is not just to prolong life at all costs
  — It is lawful to withhold CPR on the basis that to do so would be in the patient's best interests, where consideration has been given to relevant medical factors and the quality of life of patients who lack capacity
  — A competent patient has the right to accept or refuse resuscitation after he or she has been fully informed of its benefits and risks
  — It is not necessary to initiate discussion with patients if there is no reason to believe that they are likely to suffer a cardiopulmonary arrest
  — Doctors should always be prepared to discuss DNAR decisions with competent patients and they should usually consult other staff
  — However, if it is considered that CPR is unlikely to be successful, and the patient has not expressed a wish to discuss CPR, it is not always necessary or appropriate to initiate discussion with the patient to explore their wishes regarding CPR
  — If a patient wishes to receive CPR even if there is only a small chance of restarting their heart or breathing, or of prolonging their life for more than a very short period, and in spite of the risk of distressing adverse effects, doctor must provide the patient with accurate information about the nature of CPR measures procedures and the length of survival and quality of life that might realistically be expected if they were successfully resuscitated. Where a patient with capacity then requests that no DNAR decision is made in light of that discussion, doctor should respect the patient's wishes
  — Under the Human Rights Act, relatives and carers have the right to information with the consent of the competent patient. Their role is to help the doctor in decision-making and to reflect what the incompetent patient would choose in the current circumstances, if competent. They do not have the right to demand or reject resuscitation or a DNAR order
  — In case of adults who lack capacity clinician should use the guidance included in the Mental Capacity Act 2005 in assessing best interests if an individual has not made an advance decision or a lasting power of attorney (LPA).
  — The overall responsibility for decisions about CPR and DNAR rests with the consultant or general practitioner in charge of the patient's care and this may lead to dispute with the other professionals in the multidisciplinary team.

8 KEY ETHICAL AND LEGAL ISSUES IN RELATION TO CARE OF OLDER PERSONS WITH DEMENTIA

➤ In the early stages patients with dementia have the full capacity to undertake decision-making surrounding their treatment, and therefore should not be treated differently from other patients.

➤ Basic principles require the physician to tell the truth to the patient that he or she has dementia.

➤ Since there are no available preventive or therapeutic agents that can cure dementia, it is not necessary to carry out genetic testing to see if a family member has the gene or not.

➤ Any new effective treatment that is developed should be available for patients, and no one should be denied treatment solely on the grounds of cost. Any rationing should be open to public scrutiny.

➤ Patients with obvious impairment of judgement or visual–spatial difficulties should be asked to stop driving. If a person fails to take advice they should be reported to the Driver and Vehicle Licensing Agency, even if it means breaking the rule on patient confidentiality.

➤ In the later stages of the disease, doctors may have to make decisions about which treatment is best for the individual. Assessment of best interests should be performed in line with the Mental Capacity Act 2005.

➤ In end-stage dementia, artificial tube feeding is not usually appropriate and palliative care should be available when required.

➤ Restraint should only be used if it contributes to the safety of the patient or others, and should not be used for the convenience of staff.

➤ In the early stages of dementia, patients should be encouraged to consider appointing an LPA and making a valid advance decision.

➤ Patients who neglect themselves may have to be admitted to hospital under Section 47 of the National Assistance Act or moved into a residential home using Guardianship under the Mental Health Act of 1983/Mental Health Act 2007.

➤ New safeguards to prevent the deprivation of liberty will be widely applicable to the care of patients with impaired mental capacity.

9 USE OF RESTRAINTS IN OLDER PEOPLE IN HOSPITALS, NURSING HOMES AND RESIDENTIAL HOMES

➤ Restraining a competent person without consent is unlawful and constitutes a criminal assault.

➤ It is important for all individuals to have freedom of movement.

➤ The Human Rights Act 1998 and the Mental Capacity Act 2005 are relevant to the use of restraints for patients who lack capacity to consent.

➤ Human rights law informs us that restraint, although degrading at face value, is acceptable when used (proportionately) in order to treat a patient who would otherwise have to forgo beneficial treatment.

➤ Restraint, when medically necessary and used in conformity with the medical standards, has been found to be legally acceptable by the European Court of Human Rights.

➤ Section 6 of the MCA defines restraint as either the use or threat of use of force in order to undertake an action that the patient resists, or restriction of the patient's freedom of movement whether or not the patient resists.

➤ Section 11 of the MCA imposes restrictions on the lasting power of attorney in relation to use of restraint.

➤ When an incompetent patient requires medical treatment that can only be administered by using restraint, this is permissible provided:

— the form of restraint used is the least restrictive possible and used for the shortest time possible
— the treatment proposed must be in the patient's best interest
— the consequences of not treating will be seriously harmful to the patient
— restraint should be a short-term measure with the expectation of recovery
— restraint is practically possible.

➤ When an incompetent patient cannot be safely nursed without restraint, this is permissible provided:
— the form of restraint used is the least restrictive possible and used for the shortest time possible
— all other avenues of nursing without restraint have been explored
— not restraining the patient will pose a serious threat to safety of the patient or of others.

➤ In all cases where restraint is deemed necessary, assent should be sought from relatives. If the relatives refuse assent to restraint in order to administer life-prolonging treatment that the medical team believe is in the patient's best interest, a legal opinion should be sought.

➤ In all cases where restraint is believed to be necessary, the reasons why restraint is used and with whom it was discussed should be carefully documented in the patient's notes.

➤ The Deprivation of Liberty Safeguards amendment to the MCA 2005 provides procedures for authorising the deprivation of liberty of adults who lack capacity to consent to being in hospitals or care homes.

10 DEPRIVATION OF LIBERTY

➤ Specific guidance on deprivation of liberty has been produced as an addendum to the Mental Capacity Act Code of Practice.[6]

➤ The guidelines have been drafted in the light of the European Court of Human Rights judgment in the case of *HL v the United Kingdom*[7] (the Bournewood judgment).

➤ In determining deprivation of liberty, account must be taken of a range of factors such as type, duration, effects and manner of implementation of the measure that may deprive liberty.

➤ Distinction between a deprivation and restriction upon liberty is merely one of degree or intensity, and not of nature and substance.

➤ Factors that may be considered by the courts to be relevant when considering whether or not deprivation of liberty is occurring include:
— the person is not allowed to leave the facility
— the person has no or very limited choice about their life within the care home or hospital
— the person in prevented from maintaining contact with the world outside the care home or hospital.

➤ For authorisation, care homes must approach the relevant local authority and hospital must approach the Primary Care Trust.

11 ETHICAL ISSUES AROUND FEEDING

➤ A decision to artificially feed an older person requires consideration of the benefits, feasibility and morality of the proposed procedure.

➤ The Royal College of Physicians and the British Society of Gastroenterology has published a report which sets out the framework for making decisions taking into account the ethical and legal concerns.[8]

➤ The objectives of nutritional support should be evaluated by estimating the likelihood of success.

➤ The wishes and values of the patient must be considered, either contemporaneously or in the form of advance statements.

➤ For patients who are unable to express a view, a morally robust feeding decision may emerge after wider consultation in line with guidance issued in the MCA 2005.

➤ Decisions to commence feeding should be reviewed in the light of changing patient circumstances or values.

➤ Decisions to stop or to impose feeding create complex moral problems that may require legal clarification.

➤ While form of food is not considered medicine, artificial feeding, in law, is considered as part of medical treatment. Therefore, like all medical treatment it may not be administered to a competent adult without their consent.

➤ There is no obligation to give treatment that is futile or excessively burdensome.

➤ The law regards withholding or withdrawing treatment as an 'omission', not an act.

➤ In case of patients with advanced dementia, the decision whether to consider PEG should be made in the patient's best interests, using the assessment recommended by the Mental Capacity Act 2005. This should include benefits and risks associated with PEG. In relation to this decision it is important to consider the result of a large review[9] that failed to find any evidence that tube feeding prolongs survival or prevents aspiration pneumonia, reduces the risk of pressure sores or improves physical function or comfort in patients with advanced dementia.

➤ In case of patients with stroke, withdrawal of nutrition may be appropriate if patient has not improved and remains very disabled. However, when making such decisions doctors should:
— consult the patient if he/she has capacity to participate in the discussion, unless death is imminent and discussion with him/her about benefits, burdens and risks will not be appropriate.
— consult all members of the healthcare team and those close to the patient.
— seek a second expert opinion from a senior clinician who has experience of the patient's condition but is not involved in the patient's case.
— seek legal advice if significant conflicts arise between members of the healthcare team or between the healthcare team and relatives/carers.

12 DILEMMAS FACED BY DOCTORS WHEN DEALING WITH DEATH
Should a doctor tell or not tell the patient that he /she is dying?

GMC guidance is clear that doctors should share with the patient whatever they need or want to know, especially in the context of treatment decisions. Breaking bad news to a patient or his family/carer is an unwelcome task but when performed in a kind and courteous way can be rewarding. These few guidelines may help:

➤ Sit down to indicate that you have time for discussion.

➤ Try not to kill all hope, or to give too precise forecast of the duration of the illness.

➤ Do not strive for too much detachment.

➤ Undertake to continue support and relieve symptoms particularly when the symptoms are distressing and appear to affect dignity.

Is the treatment worthwhile or futile?

If the treatment is considered futile then doctor does not need to offer it to the patient. If the treatment in non-futile then doctor should offer this to the patient, if he/she is competent. If, however, the patient lacks capacity to participate in decision-making then the doctor must try to discover if there is an advance decision or an LPA. If neither exists then the decision in his/her best interests must be made using the guidance issued in the MCA Code of Practice. Here it is important to remember that euthanasia is against the law in the UK.

Should cardiopulmonary resuscitation be attempted?

While it may be considered futile to attempt CPR in a patient who is clearly dying, discussion of such decisions should be approached with sensitivity and tact, whether it is discussed within the team on the ward or relatives. If it is thought that resuscitation is likely to be successful and the individual patient still has a good quality of life, then the patient should be consulted. If the patient is not competent to take part in discussion then his/her family/carer or LPA (appointed by the patient) should be involved. At all stages it is important to stress that DNAR does not imply that the patient will not be given IV fluids or antibiotics, if required.

Whether to involve religious workers?

This is wholly dependent upon the individual's beliefs and wishes. If a person wishes to see a priest or a rabbi then all attempts should be made to fulfil his/her wish, for their involvement may alleviate suffering and preserve dignity. This may also help the family/carers with their grieving process after the patient's death.

When should active treatment be withdrawn?

When active treatment is not achieving its objective and the individual is dying, it is reasonable to stop treatment. This of course is different from the palliative care, which aims to relieve symptoms thus allowing the person to die with peace and dignity.

REFERENCES

1 Department of Health. *Mental Capacity Act 2005*. Department of Health. Available at: www.opsi.gov.uk/acts/acts2005/ukpga_20050009_en_1 (accessed 20 May 2010).
2 *Re C* (adult: refusal of treatment) (1994) 1 WLR 290.
3 *Re MB* (1997) 2 FLR 426.
4 General Medical Council. *Duties of a Doctor*. London: GMC; 2002. Available at: www.gmc-uk.org/guidance/good_medical_practice/duties_of_a_doctor.asp (accessed 20 May 2010).
5 British Medical Association. *Decisions Relating to Cardiopulmonary Resuscitation: a joint statement from the British Medical Association, the Resuscitation Council (UK), Royal College of Nursing*. London: British Medical Association; 2007.
6 Department of Constitutional Affairs. *Mental Capacity Act 2005: code of practice*. London: TSO; 2007. Available at: www.justice.gov.uk/guidance/mca-code-of-practice.htm (accessed 20 May 2010).
7 *HL v United Kingdom*. Application no. 45508/99, decision of 5 October 2005.
8 The Royal College of Physicians and the British Society of Gastroenterology. *Oral feeding difficulties and dilemmas: a guide to practical care, particularly towards the end of life*. London: Royal College of Physicians; 2010.
9 Finucane TE, Christma C, Travis K. Tube feeding in patients with advanced dementia: a review of the evidence. *JAMA*. 1999; **282**: 1365–70.

FURTHER READING

GMC. *Treatment and Care Towards the End of Life: good practice in decision making*. London: GMC; 2010. www.gmc-uk.org/End_of_life.pdf_32486688.pdf

ACKNOWLEDGEMENT

It is acknowledged that some of the information in this chapter comes from the Mental Capacity Act of Code of Practice, issued by the Lord Chancellor on 23 April 2007 in accordance with Sections 42 and 43 of the Mental Capacity Act 2005 and published by the Department for Constitutional Affairs, London, TSO (The Stationery Office).

CHAPTER 11

Elder abuse

Elder abuse or neglect (mistreatment) is a single or repeated act or lack of appropriate action occurring within any relationship where there is an expectation of trust and which causes harm or distress to an older person.

PREVALENCE
➤ Overall, 2.6% in people aged 66 and over living in private households.
➤ Women more likely than men to have experienced mistreatment.
➤ High prevalence in women aged 85 and over.
➤ Among men, abuse increases with age if neglect is excluded.
➤ Those living in rented accommodation tend to have higher prevalence.
➤ Higher prevalence in those with declining health, loneliness and depression.

AT RISK
➤ Socially isolated.
➤ Those with memory or communication difficulties.
➤ Those in a poor relationship with their carer.
➤ Those who provide housing, financial or emotional support to their carers.
➤ Carers with drug or alcohol problems.

PERPETRATORS
➤ Partner or spouse most common for neglect and interpersonal abuse.
➤ Other family members most common for financial abuse.
➤ Men more likely to abuse than women, overall, but figure is same for financial abuse.
➤ Care worker or close friend involved in a small number of cases.

TYPES OF ABUSE
➤ *physical* – hitting, pushing, slapping, inappropriate restraint, misuse of medications
➤ *sexual harassment/abuse*
➤ *neglect*
➤ *psychological* – threats of harm, threats of leaving, stopping access to other people
➤ *financial* – theft, fraud, etc.
➤ *discriminatory.*

LAW AND ABUSE
➤ There is no single law or Act that covers elder abuse.
➤ Legislation that exists to protect and therefore prevent abuse/mistreatment include:

— The National Assistance Act 1948 – *see* Chapter 9
— Social Work (Scotland) Act 1968 – *see* Chapter 9.

➤ Mental Health (care and Treatment) (Scotland) Act 2003 – replaces the Mental Health (Scotland) Act 1984 – this Act is concerned with the provision of treatment to persons with mental disorder including dementia and brain injury. It places duties on the local authorities to provide, or secure for people with mental disorders services to promote their well-being, including helping an individual who may have been exposed to ill-treatment.

➤ The National Health Service and Community Care Act 1990 – *see* Chapter 9.

➤ Mental Capacity Act 2005 and The Adults with Incapacity (Scotland) Act 2002 – both these Acts deal with management of personal, financial and medical care of individuals who lack capacity.

➤ *Criminal Law*
— Abuse that may constitute a crime includes assault, drugging, cruel and unnatural treatment, theft, rape, murder, sexual assault, incest or indecency.
— Mental Capacity Act 2005 has introduced a new criminal offence of ill-treatment or neglect of a person who lacks capacity and a person found guilty may be liable to imprisonment for a term of up to 5 years.

➤ *Civil Law*
— An abused person can bring a civil case against the abuser in relation to physical or financial abuse.

CHAPTER 12

Palliative care

HISTORY
➤ Established to improve the care of dying patients and their families.
➤ Has traditionally focused on patients with incurable cancer.
➤ Role extends to patients with non-malignant conditions.

WORLD HEALTH ORGANIZATION (WHO) DEFINES PALLIATIVE CARE AS:

Palliative care is an approach that improves the quality of life of patients and their families facing the problems associated with life-threatening illness, through the prevention and relief of suffering by means of early identification and impeccable assessment and treatment of pain and other problems, physical, psychological and spiritual.[1]

➤ Palliative care:
— provides relief from pain and other distressing symptoms
— affirms life and regards dying as a normal process
— intends neither to hasten nor postpone death
— integrates the psychological and spiritual aspects of patient care
— offers a support system to help patients live as actively as possible until death
— offers a support system to help the family cope during the patient's illness and in bereavement
— uses a team approach to address the needs of patients and their families, including bereavement counselling, if indicated
— will enhance quality of life, and may also positively influence the course of illness
— is applicable early in the course of illness, in conjunction with other therapies that prolong life, such as chemotherapy or radiation therapy, and includes those investigations needed to better understand and manage distressing clinical complications.

PRINCIPLES OF A GOOD DEATH[2]
➤ To know when death is coming and to understand what can be expected.
➤ To be able to regain control of what happens.
➤ To be afforded dignity and privacy.
➤ To have control over pain and other symptoms.
➤ To have choice and control over where death occurs.
➤ To have access to information and expertise of whatever kind is necessary.
➤ To have access to any spiritual or emotional support required.

➤ To have access to hospital care in any location, not only in hospital.
➤ To have control over who is present and who shares the end.
➤ To be able to issue advance directives to ensure wishes are respected.
➤ To have time to say goodbye and control over other aspects of timing.
➤ To be able to leave when it is time to go and not to have life prolonged pointlessly.

DELIVERY OF CARE
➤ Professionals:
  — consultants in palliative medicine
  — registrars in training
  — specialist nurses
  — general practitioners
  — district nurses
  — occupational therapists
  — physiotherapists
  — social workers
  — dieticians
  — psychologists
  — religious leaders.
➤ Informal carers:
  — family
  — friends
  — neighbours
  — volunteers.
➤ Places of care:
  — home
  — hospital
  — hospice
  — nursing/residential homes
  — respite.
➤ Communication between primary and secondary care is paramount – many patients spend some time at home during their terminal illness and may choose to die there.

CARERS
➤ Relatives, friends and neighbours often become informal carers.
➤ Burdens may be physical, psychological, social and financial.
➤ Support mechanisms include:
  — provision of knowledge (diagnosis/prognosis/symptom control)
  — emergency contact
  — practical (home modifications/aids)
  — domestic
  — psychosocial including bereavement support
  — financial (carer's allowance)
  — respite (hospice/care home/day or night-sitting services).

SYMPTOM CONTROL
Pain
➤ Common in malignancy.
➤ Multiple causes (bony/visceral/neuropathic).
➤ Understanding of pathophysiology crucial for effective management.
➤ Perception of pain affected by depression and anxiety.

➤ Pain control measures include analgesic drugs, radiotherapy, anaesthetic nerve blocks, orthopaedic surgery to stabilise long bones and replace joints, transcutaneous electrical nerve stimulation (TENS), treatment of mood disorders.

➤ Concept of 'analgesic ladder' should be employed when prescribing analgesic drugs:
— aspirin/paracetamol/non-steroidals (mild pain)
— codeine/dextropropoxyphene (moderate pain)
— morphine/other opioids (severe pain).

➤ Consider tricyclic antidepressants and anticonvulsants for neuropathic pain and bisphosphonates for bony pain.

➤ Drugs should be administered on a regular basis with adequate doses available for breakthrough symptoms.

➤ Analgesic requirements require review every 1–2 days.

➤ Remember other routes of administration if oral not possible – per rectum, subcutaneous (including syringe drivers), intravenous, intramuscular, transdermal.

Respiratory problems
Shortness of breath

➤ A manifestation of both malignant and non-malignant cardiorespiratory disease.

➤ Treatment depends on underlying cause (pleural or pericardial effusion/lung metastases/pulmonary oedema/pneumonia/pulmonary embolus).

➤ Steroids and radiotherapy are used in stridor.

➤ Anxiolytics and opioids may improve distressing symptoms.

➤ Increases carer stress.

Cough

➤ Treatment should be directed at specific cause.

➤ Consider antitussive agents such as opioids or local anaesthetic agents.

➤ Hyoscine can dry up excess secretions.

➤ Correct positioning and physiotherapy for suction and postural drainage are helpful.

Haemoptysis

➤ Treatment depends on cause – tranexamic acid and radiotherapy for tumour-related bleeds and anticoagulation for pulmonary emboli.

➤ For major haemorrhage, appropriateness of aggressive resuscitation should be reviewed – pure palliation of symptoms with analgesics and sedatives may be preferable.

Gastrointestinal complaints
Nutritional status

➤ Anorexia is common.

➤ Weight loss is a poor prognostic indicator.

➤ Cachexia associated with reduced caloric intake, malabsorption and metabolic abnormalities including release of cytokines in malignancy.

➤ Therapeutic options include nutritional supplementation and appetite stimulants.

Mouth care

➤ Commonly neglected.

➤ Oral cavity should be reviewed on a daily basis.

➤ Twice-daily brushing of teeth/dentures and tongue advised for comfort as well as hygiene.

➤ Soothe dry lips with petroleum jelly.

➤ Maintain adequate hydration.

➤ Antifungal agents such as topical nystatin or oral preparations, e.g. fluconazole, should be used to treat candidiasis.

➤ Topical anaesthetic agents ease the pain of a sore mouth.

➤ Consider topical steroids/antibiotics for aphthous ulcers.

Nausea and vomiting

➤ Culprits include drugs, hypercalcaemia, uraemia, gastric inflammation/ulceration/stasis and constipation and/or bowel obstruction.

➤ Treatment should be directed at underlying cause.

➤ Antiemetics can provide symptomatic relief – mode of action is important:
— anticholinergics, e.g. hyoscine
— antihistamines, e.g. cyclizine
— butyrophenones, e.g. haloperidol
— phenothiazines, e.g. methotrimeprazine
— prokinetics, e.g. domperidone, metoclopramide
— 5HT receptor blockers, e.g. ondansetron.

Bowel problems

➤ Constipation is a common consequence of malignancy and may be caused by:
— drugs, e.g. opioids, anticholinergics
— tumour, e.g. hypercalcaemia, spinal cord, compression, abdominopelvic disease
— general, e.g. immobility, dehydration, inaccessible toilet facilities.

➤ A combination of oral and rectal laxatives may be required.

➤ Older patients with non-malignant disease are prone to constipation with faecal impaction and overflow diarrhoea.

➤ Diarrhoea in patients with cancer is less common than constipation and may be related to drugs (e.g. laxatives, chemotherapy), radiotherapy, malabsorption and bowel obstruction.

➤ Treatment of diarrhoea should be directed at underlying cause and may necessitate use of codeine or loperamide.

Skin care

➤ Terminally ill patients at high risk of developing pressure sores.

➤ Common sites include heels, ankles, knees, buttocks, spine, elbows and shoulder blades.

➤ Predisposing factors include immobility, malnutrition, confusion, incontinence, pain, inappropriate mattresses and inadequately trained carers.

➤ Pressure areas require daily review.

➤ Risk assessment scores, e.g. Waterlow, help identify high risk patients.

➤ See Chapter 19 on pressure sores for management details.

Psychiatric problems
Delirium

➤ Older patients particularly at risk in view of impairments of hearing, vision and cognition.

➤ Other predisposing factors: drugs, including polypharmacy, electrolyte abnormalities, hypercalcaemia, sepsis.

➤ Underlying cause should be treated (sedatives may be required in some cases).

Anxiety and depression
➤ May affect both patients and carers.
➤ Effects can be physical as well as psychological.
➤ Consider psychology/psychiatry review and/or drug therapy.

Medical emergencies
Hypercalcaemia
➤ Bisphosphonate therapy for symptomatic patients and when calcium >3 mmol/L. Monthly infusions may be required to maintain normocalcaemia.

Spinal cord compression
➤ MRI investigation of choice.
➤ Treatment options include steroids, radiotherapy and/or surgery in suitable patients.

Pathological fracture
➤ Prophylactic internal fixation in selected cases.
➤ Radiotherapy may halt progression of bony metastases.

Superior vena caval obstruction
➤ Mainstay treatments are steroids and radiotherapy.

NON-MALIGNANT CONDITIONS
➤ Traditionally, palliative care has specialised in care of patients with incurable cancer.
➤ Provision of services should be on the basis of need rather than diagnosis.
➤ Other patient groups that could benefit from a palliative approach include those with chronic neurological disorders and cardiorespiratory disease.
➤ Palliative care for heart failure:
— incidence 1–2%
— increasing prevalence with age
— worse prognosis than some forms of cancer
— psychological and social morbidity
— specialist heart failure nurses could aid symptom control, reduce hospital admission rates and provide psychological support.

LIVERPOOL CARE PATHWAY (LCP, 1997)[3]
➤ An integrated care pathway designed to ensure that all dying patients (and their relatives/carers) receive a high standard of care in the last hours/days of life.
➤ Originally developed for the care of patients with cancer in the acute environment.
➤ Has been adapted for use across all care settings irrespective of diagnosis.
➤ Provides guidance on:
— symptom control
— comfort measures
— anticipatory prescribing of medication
— discontinuation of inappropriate interventions
— psychological and spiritual care
— care of the family (both before and after death of the patient).

NATIONAL CARE OF THE DYING AUDIT OF HOSPITALS (2009)[4]
➤ An audit of the use of the LCP at 155 hospitals involving 4000 patients.

➤ High standards of patient care confirmed.
➤ Key areas identified for improvement:
— communication
— spiritual care
— education and training.

END OF LIFE CARE STRATEGY (2008)[5]

➤ An initiative aiming to improve end of life care through:
— education
— communication with the palliative care team
— integrated care pathways such as the Liverpool Care Pathway.

ETHICAL ISSUES AT THE END OF LIFE
Power of attorney

➤ A patient can grant lasting power of attorney to someone trusted so that they can make decisions regarding their healthcare should there come a time when the patient is no longer able to express their wishes.

Advance directives

➤ A competent patient has the right to refuse medical treatment.
➤ Written declarations of refusal are called advance directives or 'living wills'.

Euthanasia

➤ Active voluntary euthanasia (assisted suicide) where a doctor ends a patient's life at their request is against the law in the UK.
➤ Using high doses of opiates to ease suffering may cause death (passive euthanasia) but is legal due to good intent (double effect principle).

Withholding/withdrawing life-prolonging treatment

➤ High levels of carer anxiety often surround this issue.
➤ No evidence that artificial hydration or nutrition influence survival or symptom control in dying patients – drips and nasogastric tubes could be classed as unnecessary intrusions.

Cardiorespiratory resuscitation (CPR)

➤ CPR is inappropriate if:
— there is virtually no chance of re-establishing cardiac output
— successful resuscitation would result in a quality of life unacceptable to the patient
— it is contrary to the competent patient's expressed wishes.
➤ Discussing CPR issues with palliative patients in whom resuscitation is deemed to be futile should be avoided.

BEREAVEMENT

➤ Shock leads to despair and eventually to adjustment.
➤ Support services available.

ETHNIC MINORITY GROUPS

➤ The UK is a multicultural society.
➤ Views of death and dying vary considerably between cultures.
➤ Religious needs should be respected.
➤ Healthcare professionals require training in transcultural medicine.

REFERENCES

1 World Health Organization. *Cancer: WHO definition of palliative care.* Geneva: WHO; 2006. Available at: www.who.int/cancer/palliative/definition/en (accessed 25 May 2010).

2 Debate of the Age Health and Care Study Group. *The Future of Health and Care in Older People: the best is yet to come.* London: Age Concern; 1999.

3 Ellershaw J *et al.* Developing an integrated care pathway for the dying patient. *Eur J Pall Care.* 1997; **4**(6): 203–7.

4 Marie Curie Palliative Care Institute Liverpool (MCPCIL) in collaboration with the Clinical Standards Department of the Royal College of Physicians (RCP). *National Care of the Dying Audit of Hospitals.* London: RCP; 2009. Available at: www.rcplondon.ac.uk/media/press-releases/pages/national-care-of-the-dying-audit-2009.aspx (accessed 25 May 2010).

5 Department of Health. *End of Life Care Strategy: promoting high quality care for all adults at the end of life.* London: Department of Health; 2008. Available at: www.dh.gov.uk/en/Publicationsandstatistics/Publications/PublicationsPolicyAndGuidance/DH_086277 (accessed 25 May 2010).

FURTHER READING

British Geriatrics Society. *Palliative and End of Life Care of Older People. Best practice guide.* London: British Geriatrics Society; 2009. Available at: www.bgs.org.uk/Publications/Publication%20Downloads/Comp4-8_PalliativeCare.pdf (accessed February 2009).

PART III

Clinical problems encountered in old age

CHAPTER 13

Falls

DEFINITION
➤ An event which results in a person coming to rest unintentionally on the ground or other lower level, not as a result of a major intrinsic event such as a stroke or overwhelming hazard (Tinetti *et al.* 1988).[1]

CLASSIFICATION
➤ *Faller* – someone who has fallen at least once in a given time period, e.g. 6–12 months.
➤ *Recurrent faller* – someone who has fallen twice or more during a defined time.
➤ *Once-only faller* – closely related to non-fallers.

STATISTICS
➤ A major cause of disability.
➤ The leading cause of mortality due to injury in older people over 75 years in the UK.
➤ 35–40% of community-dwelling people aged over 65 years fall annually.
➤ Rates are higher in those aged over 75 years.
➤ Incidence rates for nursing home residents and hospital inpatients are almost three times greater.
➤ 50% of fallers do so repeatedly.
➤ For previous fallers, the risk of falling again in the subsequent year is increased by two thirds.
➤ The majority of falls occur in the usual place of residence – in the home, the bedroom, kitchen and dining room are the most common settings.
➤ Indoor falls are associated with frailty, whereas outdoor events are more likely to occur in more active people.
➤ People aged under 75 years are more likely to fall outdoors than those older than 75.
➤ 80% of falls in the community occur during the day as opposed to at night.
➤ 40–60% of falls lead to injuries.
➤ Overall, injury rates are higher in institutionalised patients.

RISK FACTORS
➤ More than 400 risk factors for falling have been identified.
➤ There is often a multifactorial aetiology.
➤ The five major categories cover the following:
1   Environmental
     • loose carpets and rugs

- steep stairs
- poor lighting
- slippery floors
- poorly fitting footwear and clothes
- lack of safety equipment, e.g. grab rails
- inaccessible lights or windows.

2 Drugs
- alcohol
- analgesics
- antiarrhythmics
- antidepressants
- antihistamines
- antihypertensives
- antipsychotics
- sedatives
- polypharmacy (more than four drugs).

3 Medical conditions
- arthritis
- cognitive impairment
- depression
- parkinsonism
- postural hypotension
- previous falls
- stroke
- visual impairment.

4 Nutritional factors
- calcium and vitamin D deficiency.

5 Exercise
- lack of exercise.

CONSEQUENCES
Injury
- ➤ 40–60% of falls lead to injury
- ➤ 30–50% are minor
- ➤ 5–6% are major (excluding fracture)
- ➤ 5% result in fracture.

Hospital admission
- ➤ Admission rates due to falls are six times higher in people aged over 85 years compared to those in the 65 to 69-year-old age group.

Psychological
- ➤ A third of those aged over 60 years develop a fear of falling.
- ➤ Loss of confidence.
- ➤ Post-fall anxiety.
- ➤ Self-imposed functional limitation.
- ➤ Social isolation.
- ➤ Depression.

Disability
- ➤ Subsequent dependency.

Long lie

➤ Hypothermia.
➤ Pressure sores.
➤ Dehydration.
➤ Rhabdomyolysis.
➤ Bronchopneumonia.

Institutionalisation

➤ Fall-related accidents are predisposing factors in 40% of events leading to long-term care in older people.

NATIONAL SERVICE FRAMEWORK FOR OLDER PEOPLE: STANDARD 6: FALLS (2001)[2]

Aims

➤ To reduce the number of falls that result in serious injury.
➤ To ensure effective treatment and rehabilitation.
➤ To provide advice on prevention through a specialised falls service.

Prevention

Population approach

➤ Public health strategies:
  — physical activity
  — healthy eating
  — reduced smoking.
➤ Environmental strategies:
  — clear pavements
  — street lighting.
➤ Information provision:
  — leaflets.

Individual approach

➤ Targeting risk factors.

Specialised falls service

➤ Older people who fall should be referred if any of the following apply:
  — previous fragility fracture
  — emergency department attendance with a fall
  — ambulance called after a fall
  — two or more intrinsic risk factors and a fall
  — frequent unexplained falls
  — unsafe housing conditions
  — fear of falling.

Intervention

➤ Diagnosis and treatment of medical problems.
➤ Physiotherapy and occupational therapy assessment.
➤ Equipment to improve home safety.
➤ Social care support.

Rehabilitation

➤ The aims of rehabilitation are to:
  — improve stability during standing, transferring and walking through:

- balance training
- muscle strengthening
- improving flexibility
- providing appropriate safety equipment.
— regain independence and confidence
— modify the home environment and remove hazards
— teach strategies to cope with further falls
— establish a network of community support if required.

Long-term support
➤ Pendant alarms.
➤ Personal or domestic services.
➤ Social activities.
➤ Monitoring of needs.

Falls service
➤ All hospital trusts should have an established falls service.
➤ Local policies for referral should be developed.
➤ Members of the team should include:
  — consultants in geriatrics
  — nurses
  — physiotherapists
  — occupational therapists
  — social workers
  — pharmacists
  — podiatrists.
➤ Access to the following professionals should be available:
  — dieticians
  — optometrists
  — orthotists
  — ophthalmologists
  — audiologists
  — health advocates.
➤ *See* Figure 13.1 Falls care pathway.

HIP PROTECTORS
➤ Advocated as a means of reducing the risk of hip fracture following a fall.
➤ Reduce the force transmitted to the proximal femur through the greater trochanter.
➤ Two types: energy-absorbing padding; semi-rigid plastic shield.
➤ Should be used at all times when at risk of falling (including at night).
➤ Problems with adherence especially in community settings (uncomfortable/unsightly/difficult to get on and off).
➤ Cost £40 a pair (each user ideally needs 3 pairs).
➤ Evidence suggests that hip protectors can reduce the incidence of hip fracture in high risk older people in institutional care and in highly motivated community dwellers.

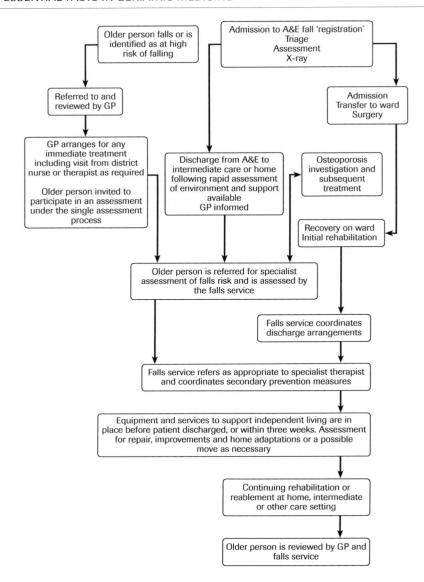

FIGURE 13.1 Falls care pathway (NSF).

REFERENCES

1 Tinetti ME *et al.* Risk factors for falls among elderly persons living in the community. *N Engl J Med.* 1988; **319**: 1701–7.

2 Department of Health. *National Service Framework for Older People.* London: Department of Health; 2001. www.dh.gov.uk

FURTHER READING

British Geriatrics Society. *Best Practice Guide: falls.* London: BGS; 2007. www.bgs.org.uk
National Institute for Health and Clinical Excellence. *The assessment and prevention of falls in older people. NICE guideline 21.* London: NIHCE; 2004. www.nice.org.uk/cg21

CHAPTER 14

Dizziness

Dizziness is a common symptom in older people occurring in up to 30% of patients over 65. Symptoms can range from mild and brief to severe and disabling. It is important to enquire as to exactly what the patient means by dizziness to help determine the underlying cause. There are three main types of dizziness:
➤ Vertigo.
➤ Presyncope.
➤ Disequilibrium.

Occasionally, patients report blurred vision, feelings of unreality, or blackouts and these symptoms need to be investigated appropriately.

COMMON CAUSES OF DIZZINESS IN THOSE OVER 65
➤ Benign paroxysmal positional vertigo (BPPV).
➤ Cervical spondylosis.
➤ Anxiety or hyperventilation.
➤ Poor vision.
➤ Postural hypotension.
➤ Arrhythmias.

Patients with dizziness often have difficulty describing their symptoms so determining the cause can be challenging. A good history followed by cardiological, neurological and locomotor examination, and simple provocation tests (e.g. Hallpike manoeuvre, postural blood pressure measurement) may help define the cause. The first step in assessing the patient with dizziness is establishing whether the patient has vertigo versus another type of dizziness.

DIAGNOSTIC CRITERIA THAT HELP DIFFERENTIATE SOME COMMON CAUSES OF DIZZINESS
➤ *BPPV* – brief episodes of vertigo on change of position (Hallpike manoeuvre – see p. 86).
➤ *Cervical spondylosis* – symptoms on neck movement with reduced range of movement of cervical spine.
➤ *Postural hypotension* – symptoms relate to change in posture – from supine or sitting to standing with significant drop in systolic blood pressure (>20 mmHg).
➤ *Central vascular disease* – multiple white matter lesions (periventricular leukomalacia) are an important source of unsteadiness with abnormal gait and increased tone.

Vertigo is a specific type of dizziness described as a sensation of spinning or swaying when the body is stationary. It results from a problem with the inner ear balance mechanism (vestibular system), the brain or the connections between the two. It may be

➤ *Subjective* – the person has a false sensation of movement (most common)
➤ *Objective* – surroundings move past a persons' field of vision

DIFFERENTIAL DIAGNOSIS OF VERTIGO IN OLDER PEOPLE

There are many causes of vertigo and they are usually subclassified into peripheral and central causes (*see* Table 14.1). The common causes in older people are shown in Table 14.1.

In determining whether a patient has a central or peripheral cause of vertigo, key information from the history that is helpful includes:

➤ The timing and duration of vertigo – the longer the duration the more likely a central cause.
➤ Aggravating or provoking factors – e.g. change in head position, head injury.
➤ Associated symptoms especially neurological, hearing loss, tinnitus, headache, nausea and vomiting.
➤ Medication history (*see* Table 14.1).

Physical examination, with particular attention to head and neck, cardiovascular and neurological systems, hearing and diagnostic provocation tests, is essential.

The Hallpike manoeuvre, described by Dix and Hallpike, is the most useful provocative test. In this test, a person is brought from sitting to a supine position, with the head turned 45 degrees to one side and extended about 20 degrees backward. It can be used to confirm the diagnosis of benign paroxysmal positional vertigo (BPPV) with a positive predictive value of 83%. The classic nystagmus of BPPV occurs when the head is reclined and turned to the affected side and the intensity of symptoms wanes with repeated manoeuvres. A purely vertical or torsional nystagmus with a latency of less than 5 seconds that does not wane with repeated manoeuvres suggests a central cause.

Key distinguishing features of peripheral versus central causes of vertigo are listed in Table 14.2.

Laboratory tests are rarely helpful in identifying the cause of vertigo.

Indications for neuroimaging include:

➤ neurological signs and symptoms
➤ risk factors for cerebrovascular disease
➤ progressive unilateral hearing loss.

Magnetic resonance imaging (MRI) is usually considered more appropriate that computed tomography (CT) because of its superiority in visualising the posterior fossa. Magnetic resonance or conventional angiography may be useful in diagnosing vascular causes such as vertebrobasilar insufficiency.

Treatment of vertigo depends on the underlying cause.

➤ BPPV may be treated with vestibular rehabilitation (Brandt-Daroff exercises) or the Epley manoeuvre.
➤ Betahistine (histamine analogue) and or a mild diuretic (dyazide) may help reduce frequency of attacks in Ménière's disease.
➤ Antihistamines and phenothiazines may be useful in acute attacks of Ménière's disease and vestibular neuronitis.
➤ Gentamicin injections through the eardrum have recently been shown to be useful in Ménière's disease.
➤ Patients with Ramsay Hunt syndrome should be treated with an anti-herpetic agent and prednisolone 60 mg daily for 10 days.

TABLE 14.1 Differential diagnosis of vertigo in older people

Cause	Description
Peripheral causes	
Benign positional paroxysmal vertigo (BPPV)	Transient episodes (usually seconds) of vertigo on head movement caused by stimulation of vestibular sense organs by canaloliathiasis
Acute vestibular neuronitis	Sudden onset of severe vertigo very sensitive to head movements, associated with nausea and vomiting and lasting a few days. Due to inflammation of the vestibular nerve caused by viral infection. Vertigo and disequilibrium on head movement may persist for weeks to months
Herpes zoster oticus (Ramsay Hunt syndrome)	Vesicular eruption affecting the ear due to reactivation of varicella – zoster virus
Ménière's disease	Recurrent episodes of vertigo, hearing loss, and tinnitus (usually 5–15 minutes) occurring spontaneously. Due to increased volume of endolymph in the semi-circular canals. Permanent hearing loss and balance problems often occur in the long term
Central causes	
Cerebrovascular disease (stroke or transient ischaemic attack, TIA)	Isolated dizziness almost never reflects a TIA or stroke. The only stroke commonly associated with dizziness is lateral medullary infarction due to occlusion of the posterior inferior cerebellar artery resulting from vertebral artery thrombosis. There is often associated nausea and vomiting and additional neurological signs such as nystagmus, ptosis, facial pain and contralateral sensory loss, dysarthria, dysphasia and ataxia
Cerebellopontine angle tumour	Acoustic neuroma, brainstem glioma
Vertebrobasilar migrane	Episodic vertigo and headache often with aura and accompanied by vomiting, photophobia or phonophobia
Other causes	
Cervical vertigo (sometimes called top-shelf vertigo)	Triggered by somatosensory input from head and neck movements
Drug-induced	Adverse reaction to aminoglycosides, anticonvulsants, alcohol, antidepressants, antihypertensives, diuretics, salicylates, quinine, sedatives and hyponotics
Carbon – monoxide poisoning	
Para-neoplastic syndrome	Vertigo-like symptoms may appear in the form of the opsoclonus myoclonus syndrome – a multi-faceted neurological disorder associated with cancer

➤ Patients with cerebrovascular disease should be prescribed aspirin, statins and have their blood pressure controlled according to guidelines.
➤ Vestibular rehabilitation may also be helpful in older patients with vestibular neuronitis whose symptoms don't recover quickly and in drug induced vertigo.

Further assessment of the patient with non-vertigenous dizziness depends on the type of symptoms described.

TABLE 14.2 Characteristics to distinguish between peripheral and central causes of vertigo

Characteristic	Peripheral	Central
Nystagmus	Combined horizontal and torsional, inhibited by fixation of eyes onto object, does not change direction with gaze to either side, fades after a few days	Purely vertical, horizontal or torsional, not inhibited by fixation of eyes onto object, may change direction with gaze towards fast phase, may last weeks to months
Imbalance	Mild to moderate – able to walk	Severe – unable to stand or walk
Nausea and vomiting	May be severe	Varies
Hearing loss and tinnitus	Common	Rare
Non-auditory neurological symptoms	Rare	Common
Latency following provocative diagnostic manoeuvre	Long – up to 20 seconds	Short – up to 5 seconds

THE PATIENT WITH PRESYNCOPE

Patients usually describe a feeling of light-headedness, visual dimming or blurring, generalised weakness and a sense of 'going down' or imminent loss of consciousness but without the actual physical rotary motion described with vertigo. Like syncope it is usually due to a critical fall in systemic perfusion pressure and is usually either cardiogenic or situational.

Common causes of cardiogenic presyncope in older people

➤ Bradyarrhythmias (*see* Chapter 29).
➤ Tachyarrhythmias (*see* Chapter 29).
➤ Obstruction to cardiac outflow – aortic stenosis and hypertrophic cardiomyopathy.
➤ Pulmonary stenosis, pulmonary hypertension and pulmonary embolism.

Assessment and investigation of the patient with possible cardiogenic presyncope

➤ Accurate history of symptoms and circumstances and witness account, if available.
➤ Physical examination – pulse and presence of murmurs.
➤ Resting ECG – if physical examination and resting ECG are normal there is low yield from further cardiac investigation. Think about situational presyncope.
➤ Echocardiogram if indicated after physical examination.
➤ Prolonged cardiac monitoring. If 24-hour and 7-day Holter monitoring do not capture an event an implantable loop recorder may be indicated.

Common causes of situation presyncope in older people

Situational presyncope occurs in circumstances that provide a logical explanation for falls in systemic perfusion pressure and the diagnosis is usually possible after a careful history.

Factors contributing to situation presyncope and syncope include:
➤ Micturition – usually older men and passing large volumes of urine at night.
➤ Defecation – associated with straining.

➤ Volume depletion.
➤ Cough – usually associated with prolonged spasms of coughing in patients with respiratory disease. A posterior fossa mass can cause syncope after a single cough.
➤ Post-prandial syndrome – occurs in older people and is thought to be due to increased blood flow to the GI vasculature and an inability to compensate haemodynamically.
➤ *Orthostatic hypotension* is defined as a drop in systolic pressure of greater than 20 mmHg on moving from supine to upright position. Symptoms are unusual unless pressure fall below 100 mmHg systolic. Causes include a small fibre autonomic poly neuropathy (e.g diabetes mellitus, amyloid), degeneration of sympathetic neurones in the intermediate zone of the spinal cord such as in Parkinson's or multi-system degenerative disease (Shy-Drager syndrome), drugs (diuretics, antihypertensives, antidepressants and neuroleptics). Treatment is largely supportive with advice on avoiding precipitating factors, medication review and increasing fluid and salt intake. Pharmacological therapy with fludrocortisone and or midodrine may be helpful in severely symptomatic patients.
➤ *Carotid sinus syndrome* is defined as asystole >3 seconds (cardioinhibitory) or a fall of >50 mmHg in systolic blood pressure (vasodepressor) elicited by carotid sinus massage in the supine or tilted position. Cardiac pacing is beneficial in the cardioinhibitory type. Vasodepressor symptoms may respond to midodrine.
➤ *Neurocardiogenic syncope* is characterised by the development of presyncopal symptoms over several minutes followed by syncope if the patient does not lie down. Patients typically appear pale and diaphoretic. It is usually due to stimulation of left ventricular mechanoreceptors leading to hypotension. The diagnosis is usually made on basis of the typical history and can be confirmed by head-up tilt testing. Avoiding precipitating circumstances and advice to lie down as soon as symptoms start is usually all that is required.
➤ *Vasovagal syncope* is similar to the above but more common in young patients and due to increased vagus-nerve efferent output with resulting bradycardia. It is typically precipitated by prolonged standing or stressful situations.

THE PATIENT WITH DISEQUILIBRIUM

Disequilibrium is characterised by unsteadiness on the feet usually with no cranial sensation and often associated with a fear of falling.

It usually reflects neurological disease involving the parasagital region of the cerebrum, the basal ganglia, cerebellum, brainstem spinal cord or peripheral nerves.

Small vessel disease is the most frequent finding but neoplasms, hyprocephalus, subdural haematoma, neurodegenerative disease and peripheral neuropathy may be responsible.

Neurological examination will usually provide localising clues so that a circumscribed diagnostic work-up can be designed.

Multifactorial disequilibrium syndrome (MDS) is the commonest cause of disequilibrium in older people. Input from several sensory systems is essential to maintain balance.
➤ Vestibular input from the labyrinths via the vestibular nerves.
➤ Vision especially if there is substantial disparity between the two eyes.
➤ Somatosensory input particularly from position receptors in the ankle (affected by peripheral neuropathy, posterior column disease or cervical myelopathy).

Other non-neurological abnormalities that can affect balance include:
➤ pain and limited range of movement due to arthritis

➤ altered centre of gravity due to leg shortening or scoliosis
➤ deconditioning.

The act of walking also requires the coordinated function of several sub-systems in the central nervous system.

➤ The spinal cord defines the reciprocal movement of the legs.
➤ The brainstem and cerebellum link this movement to the antigravity muscles and modify it on basis of vestibular and somatosensory input.
➤ The midline cerebrum defines the context of walking with respect to external circumstances (e.g when to start and stop) and with respect to other movement (e.g stepping up or over).

Patients with MDS have defects in several of these systems and the central nervous systems supporting balance.

Most commonly, patients have small vessel ischaemic damage due to microvascular disease but stroke, Parkinson's and cerebellar degeneration due to alcohol abuse may be contributing factors.

Classically, these patients have a reduced stride, broad base, feel unsteady and maintain one or both hands in contact with walls or furniture. They often have difficulty initiating walking and turning and may fall frequently.

Brain imaging (MRI or CT) and laboratory studies for polyneuropathy should be performed. Spinal cord imaging is only required if there are localising signs.

Management involves correction of visual impairment, gait therapy, provision of aids and adaptations

RECOMMENDED READING

European Society of Cardiology. Guidelines for the diagnosis and management of syncope (version 2009). *Eur Heart J.* 2009; **30**: 2631–71.

CHAPTER 15

Osteoporosis and fractures

DEFINITION
➤ Osteoporosis can be defined as:
  — A progressive systemic skeletal disease characterised by low bone mass and microarchitectural deterioration of bone tissue with a consequent increase in bone fragility and susceptibility to fracture.
  — Bone with a density below the mean value for a young adult by >2.5 standard deviations as determined by DEXA scanning.[1]
➤ A fragility fracture:
  — Results from a fall from standing height or less.
  — Is a strong independent risk factor for further fracture and may be regarded as an indication for treatment without the need for bone mineral density measurement when the clinical history is unequivocal.

BONE PATHOLOGY
➤ Three types of cells are involved in the continuous process of bone remodelling:
  — osteoclasts: resorb bone
  — osteoblasts: synthesise bone matrix
  — osteocytes: mature osteoblasts that maintain extracellular components of bone.
➤ Bone loss occurs if resorption exceeds formation. Peak bone mass is attained by 30 years of age.

STATISTICS
➤ 30% of women aged over 80 have osteoporosis.
➤ 1 in 3 women and 1 in 12 men sustain osteoporotic fractures.
➤ More than 200 000 osteoporotic fractures are diagnosed in UK each year.
➤ Wrist, hip and spine are the most commonly affected sites.
➤ Other sites include proximal humerus, pelvis and lower limb.
➤ Hip fractures alone account for >20% of orthopaedic bed occupancy.
➤ Hip fracture costs the NHS £1.7 billion each year.
➤ Devastating consequences of hip fracture:[2]
  — 20% 12-month mortality
  — 50% fail to return to independent living at one year
  — 40% are unable to walk independently
  — 60% have difficulty with at least one essential ADL
  — 80% are restricted in other activities, e.g. driving, shopping
  — 27% enter a nursing home for the first time.
➤ Osteoporosis remains underdetected and undertreated in older people.

RISK FACTORS
➤ Untreated hypogonadism (premature menopause/secondary amenhorrhoea/ primary hypogonadism in women/primary or secondary hypogonadism in men).
➤ Glucocorticoid therapy.
➤ Other drugs (e.g. anticonvulsants/heparin/lithium/thyroxine over-replacement).
➤ Chronic disease (e.g. hyperparathyroidism/hyperthyroidism/liver disease).
➤ Radiological osteopenia.
➤ Family history.
➤ Reduced calcium and vitamin D intake.
➤ Smoking.
➤ Excess alcohol.
➤ Prolonged immobility.
➤ Caucasian.
➤ Additional risk factors for fracture:
  — previous fragility fracture (increases the risk for further fracture two-fold)
  — recurrent falls
  — low body mass index.

CLINICAL FEATURES
➤ Usually asymptomatic until fractures occur.
➤ Back pain secondary to vertebral crush fractures.
➤ Thoracic kyphosis resulting in loss of height.

INVESTIGATION OF FRAGILITY FRACTURE
➤ If clinically indicated, appropriate simple tests to exclude other pathology, for example:
  — myeloma (FBC/ESR/serum electrophoresis/urinary Bence Jones protein)
  — bony metastases (calcium/LFTs)
  — spinal X-rays may reveal lytic/sclerotic lesions.
➤ Premenopausal women and men with osteoporosis should undergo specialist assessment to determine cause.
➤ Consider DEXA scanning.

DUAL ENERGY X-RAY ABSORPTIOMETRY (DEXA)
➤ High specificity but low sensitivity for predicting future fracture risk.
➤ Not suitable as a population screening tool.
➤ May be useful in monitoring bone loss, assessing effect of treatment and avoiding inappropriate therapy.

FRACTURE RISK ASSESSMENT TOOL (FRAX) 2008[3]
➤ An online tool that predicts 10-year fracture risk.
➤ Can be used for primary and secondary fracture prevention.

UK GUIDELINES FOR PRIMARY AND SECONDARY PREVENTION OF OSTEOPOROTIC FRAGILITY FRACTURES
National Institute for Health and Clinical Excellence (2008)[4,5]
National Osteoporosis Guideline Group (2008)[6]
➤ Both sets of guidelines have a number of shortcomings.
➤ Clinical judgement should not be overridden.
➤ Key recommendation by both groups:
  — older female patients (NICE aged 75 years and above/NOGG postmenopausal)

with a history of fragility fracture should be treated without the need for further evaluation (i.e. DEXA scan is not necessary).

MANAGEMENT OF OSTEOPOROSIS
Exclude secondary causes
➤ Especially in men where secondary causes are found in up to 60% of cases.

Lifestyle advice
➤ Adequate dietary intake of calcium and vitamin D.
➤ Regular weight-bearing exercise.
➤ Avoidance of excess alcohol and tobacco.
➤ Falls prevention.

Hip protectors
➤ *See* Chapter 13 on falls.

Pharmacological interventions
Bisphosphonates
➤ Inhibit activation and function of osteoclasts.
➤ May directly stimulate formation of bone by osteoblasts.
➤ Poor oral absorption requires them to be taken on an empty stomach with a glass of water, the patient remaining upright for 30 minutes to reduce risk of oesophageal irritation.
➤ Side effects include oesophageal ulceration/stricture, constipation and renal impairment.
➤ Generic alendronate prescribed weekly is recommended as first line therapy in most guidelines.
➤ Intravenous bisphosphonates (such as ibandronate and zolendronate) can be considered in cases of intolerance of alendronate or other agents or where poor compliance is an issue.

Strontium
➤ Acts primarily as an anti-resorptive agent.
➤ May also produce an anabolic effect.
➤ Should be taken 2 hours after food to optimise absorption (usually prescribed at night).
➤ Associated with a small risk of venous thromboembolism.

Teriparatide
➤ Recombinant parathyroid hormone.
➤ In low doses exerts an anabolic effect as opposed to high dose parathyroid hormone.
➤ Subcutaneous administration.
➤ Costly.

Raloxifene
➤ A selective estrogen receptor modulator.
➤ Potential side effects include hot flushes, leg oedema and thromboembolism.
➤ Has not yet demonstrated reduced fracture incidence at the hip and so is generally used second line.

Calcium and vitamin D

➤ For patients:
— likely to be deficient in vitamin D but not in need of anti-resorptive therapy
— prescribed anti-resorptive drugs.
➤ Especially useful in frail, housebound older people and residential/nursing home residents.

Hormone replacement therapy

➤ Recent trial data on HRT has lead the Committee on Safety of Medicines to strongly recommend that it no longer be used in the prevention and treatment of osteoporosis.

Osteoporosis in men

➤ Underrecognised and undertreated.
➤ 20% of men aged over 50 years will sustain a fragility fracture.
➤ 30% of hip fractures and 20% of vertebral fractures occur in men.
➤ Mortality rates are higher in men with fracture than in women.
➤ Alendronate, risedronate and teriparatide are all licensed for use.
➤ Secondary causes should be identified and referred for specialty opinion if necessary.

NATIONAL SERVICE FRAMEWORK FOR OLDER PEOPLE (2001)[7]

➤ Osteoporosis is a target area for improvement in Standard Six: Falls (*see* Chapter 13 on falls).

THE CARE OF PATIENTS WITH FRAGILITY FRACTURE (BRITISH ORTHOPAEDIC ASSOCIATION'S 'BLUE BOOK' 2007)[8]

➤ Key elements of good care include:
— prompt admission to orthopaedic care
— rapid comprehensive assessment: medical, surgical and anaesthetic
— minimal delay to surgery
— accurate and well-performed surgery
— prompt mobilisation
— early multidisciplinary rehabilitation
— early supported discharge and ongoing community rehabilitation
— secondary prevention combining bone protection and falls assessment.
➤ Six standards for hip fracture care:
— all patients with hip fracture should be admitted to an acute orthopaedic ward within 4 hours of presentation
— all patients with hip fracture who are medically fit should have surgery within 48 hours of admission, and during normal working hours
— all patients with hip fracture should be assessed and cared for with a view to minimising their risk of developing a pressure ulcer
— all patients presenting with a fragility fracture should be managed on an orthopaedic ward with routine access to acute orthogeriatric medical support from the time of admission
— all patients presenting with a fragility fracture should be assessed to determine their need for antiresorptive therapy to prevent future osteoporotic fractures
— all patients presenting with a fragility fracture following a fall should be offered multidisciplinary assessment and intervention to prevent future falls.
➤ An orthogeriatrician should be fully integrated in the work of the fracture service.

➤ A Fracture Liaison Service (FLS) delivered by a specialist nurse should be considered in all units (*see* Figure 15.1 below).

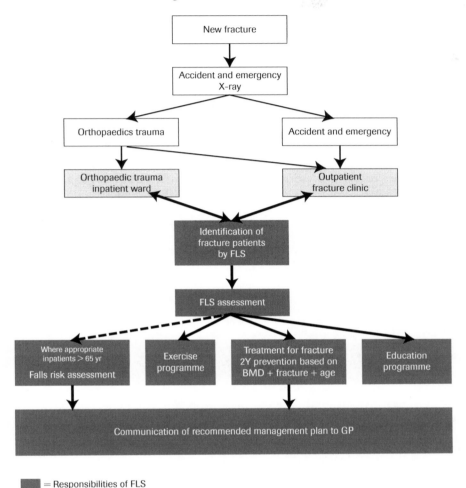

= Responsibilities of FLS

FIGURE 15.1 Fracture Liaison Service (FLS).

NATIONAL CLINICAL AUDIT OF FALLS AND BONE HEALTH IN OLDER PEOPLE (2007)[9]

➤ Examines the clinical services available for older people who have fallen and sustained fragility fractures.
➤ Widespread deficiencies in care provision have been identified:
 — 31% of operations for hip fracture are delayed beyond the 48 hour target, increasing mortality rates
 — most patients discharged home from Accident and Emergency following a fall are not offered a falls risk assessment and only 22% are referred for exercise training to reduce the risk of further falls
 — after 3 months only one fifth of these patients are on appropriate treatment for osteoporosis

— even after recovering from hip fracture surgery less than 50% are on appropriate osteoporosis treatment
— for the minority of patients who attend a falls clinic the falls and fracture risk assessments and treatment offered are better.

➤ Recommendations include commissioning a patient care pathway for the secondary prevention of falls and fractures.

NATIONAL HIP FRACTURE DATABASE[10]

➤ The Clinical Effectiveness and Evaluation Unit of the Royal College of Physicians is working with the British Geriatrics Society and the British Orthopaedic Association to establish a national hip fracture registry.

➤ The proposal is to collect a standardised dataset on all patients admitted with hip fracture in the UK.

➤ The data would reflect hip fracture management and secondary prevention for falls and osteoporosis.

➤ This information could be used for monitoring performance and benchmarking of practice.

REFERENCES

1 World Health Organization. *Assessment of Fracture Risk and its Application to Screening for Postmenopausal Osteoporosis: report of the World Health Organization Study Group.* WHO Technical Report Series No. 843. Geneva: World Health Organization; 1994.

2 Cooper C. The crippling consequences of fractures and their impact on quality of life. *Am J Med.* 1997; **103**: 125–75.

3 World Health Organization. *Collaborating Centre for Metabolic Bone Diseases. FRAX: WHO Fracture Risk Assessment Tool.* University of Sheffield; 2008. Available at: www.shef.ac.uk/FRAX (accessed 25 May 2010).

4 National Institute for Health and Clinical Excellence. *Alendronate, etidronate, risedronate, raloxifene and strontium ranelate for the primary prevention of osteoporotic fragility fractures in postmenopausal women.* NICE Technology appraisal guidance 160. London: NIHCE; 2008. Available at: www.nice.org.uk/ta160 (accessed 25 May 2010).

5 National Institute for Health and Clinical Excellence. *Alendronate, etidronate, risedronate, raloxifene, strontium ranelate and teriparatide for the secondary prevention of osteoporotic fragility fractures in postmenopausal women. NICE technology appraisal guidance 161.* London: NIHCE; 2008. Available at: www.nice.org.uk/ta161 (accessed 25 May 2010).

6 National Osteoporosis Guideline Group. *Osteoporosis: clinical guideline for prevention and treatment: executive summary.* Sheffield: NOGG; 2008. Available at: www.iofbonehealth.org/download/osteofound/filemanager/iof/csa/consensus-guidelines/nogg-executive-summary.pdf (accessed 25 May 2010).

7 Department of Health. *National Service Framework for Older People.* London: Department of Health; 2001. Available at: www.dh.gov.uk/en/publicationsandstatistics/publications/publicationspolicyandguidance/dh_4003066 (accessed 26 May 2010).

8 British Orthopaedic Association. *The Care of Patients with Fragility Fracture* (The Blue Book). London: British Orthopaedic Association; 2007. Available at: www.fractures.com/pdf/BOA-BGS-Blue-Book.pdf (accessed 25 May 2010).

9 The Clinical Effectiveness and Evaluation Unit. *National Clinical Audit of Falls and Bone Health in Older People.* London: Royal College of Physicians; 2007. Available at: www.rcplondon.ac.uk/clinical-standards/ceeu/documents/fbhop-national report.pdf (accessed 25 May 2010).

10 National Hip Fracture Database. www.nhfd.co.uk

CHAPTER 16

Musculoskeletal disorders

OSTEOARTHRITIS
Definition
➤ Osteoarthritis is a clinical syndrome of joint pain associated with functional limitation and reduced quality of life.

Statistics
➤ A leading cause of pain and disability worldwide.
➤ The most common form of arthritis.
➤ Up to 8.5 million people in the UK are affected.
➤ Most common sites include hands, feet, knees, hips and spine.
➤ More than 120 000 joint replacements are performed in the UK each year.

Predisposing factors
➤ Genetics.
➤ Increasing age.
➤ Female gender.
➤ Obesity.
➤ History of trauma.
➤ Previous joint inflammation or infection.

Pathology
➤ Localised loss of articular cartilage.
➤ Remodelling of adjacent bone leading to osteophyte formation.

Clinical features
➤ Morning joint stiffness of less than 30 minutes.
➤ Joint pain exacerbated by use.
➤ Crepitus/bony swelling ± joint effusion.

Radiological findings
➤ Loss of joint space.
➤ Osteophyte formation.
➤ Subchondral bone thickening.
➤ Cyst formation.

NICE Guidance on care and management (2008)[1]
Assessment
➤ Assessment should:

— be holistic
— review function and gait
— involve examination of joints above and below those affected
— establish effect on quality of life
— exclude mood disorder
— characterise care needs
— ascertain severity of joint pain.

General management
➤ Promotion of health and well-being.
➤ Reduction of risk factors.
➤ Patient-centred approach.

Non-pharmacological management
➤ Exercise.
➤ Manipulation and stretching.
➤ Weight loss where appropriate.
➤ Transcutaneous electrical nerve stimulation (TENS).
➤ Appropriate footwear.
➤ Consideration of braces/supports/insoles.
➤ Assistive devices such as walking aids, tap turners.

Pharmacological management
➤ Paracetamol ± topical non-steroidal anti-inflammatory drugs (NSAIDs) should be considered before oral NSAIDs, COX-2 (cyclooxygenase) inhibitors or opioids.
➤ Intra-articular steroid injections can be considered for moderate/severe pain.

Surgical intervention
➤ Consider when symptoms are refractory to non-surgical treatment and impacting negatively on quality of life.
➤ Refer before severe pain and functional limitation develop.
➤ Age alone should not be a barrier.

Specific management issues relating to age
➤ Symptoms of comorbid conditions may limit adherence to an exercise programme.
➤ Patients may be intolerant of analgesic agents.
➤ Treatment choices (including surgery) may be restricted by other medical conditions.

RHEUMATOID ARTHRITIS
Definition
➤ Rheumatoid arthritis is a chronic, progressive autoimmune disease associated with inflammation mainly in synovial joints.

Statistics
➤ Affects more than 400 000 people in the UK.
➤ More common in women.
➤ Peak prevalence is 35–65 years.

Clinical features
- Joint pain and swelling.
- Morning joint stiffness for more than one hour.
- Symmetrical distribution.
- Small joints of hands and feet usually affected initially.

Extra-articular manifestations
- Present in 30% of cases.
- Rheumatoid factor positive.
- *Skin* – nodules/vasculitis/palmar erythema.
- *Eyes* – episcleritis/scleritis/scleromalacia.
- *Blood* – anaemia/neutropenia/thrombocytosis.
- *Heart* – pericarditis/increased cardiovascular risk.
- *Lungs* – pleurisy/fibrosis.
- *Kidneys* – amyloidosis.
- *Nerves* – peripheral neuropathy/mononeuritis multipex.

Diagnosis
- Clinical findings.
- Rheumatoid factor is positive in 70% of cases.
- ESR/CRP reflect disease activity.
- X-rays.

Radiological findings
- May be normal in early disease.
- Abnormalities include:
  — soft tissue swelling
  — loss of joint space
  — bony erosions
  — subluxation
  — juxta-articular osteopaenia.

NICE Guidance on management (2009)[2]
Key messages
- Early diagnosis and referral to specialist care.
- Early intensive treatment of active disease.

General management
- Patient education.
- Information on support groups, e.g. National Rheumatoid Arthritis Society.[3]

Pharmacological management
- Caution with NSAIDs and COX 2 inhibitors in older people.
- Disease-modifying drugs should be commenced within 3 months of onset of persistent symptoms, e.g. methotrexate.
- Short courses of steroids may be required for flare-ups.
- Biological therapies such as TNF (tumour necrosis factor) α-blockers, e.g. infliximab.

Multidisciplinary input
- Physiotherapy.
- Occupational therapy.

➤ Podiatry.
➤ Psychology.
➤ Specialist nurse.

Surgical referral
➤ Consider in the following circumstances:
  — persistent pain despite optimal non-surgical therapy
  — worsening joint function
  — progressive deformity
  — imminent or actual tendon rupture
  — nerve compression
  — stress fracture
  — cervical myelopathy.

Annual review
➤ Assess disease activity and joint damage.
➤ Ascertain functional abilities.
➤ Determine effect on quality of life and screen for depression.
➤ Look for evidence of extra-articular disease.
➤ Optimise medication.
➤ Make appropriate multidisciplinary referrals.
➤ Consider the need for surgical review.

GOUT
Definition
➤ Gout is characterised by acute, self-limiting attacks of arthritis secondary to intra-articular precipitation of monosodium urate crystals.

Statistics
➤ More common in men.
➤ Prevalence 7% in men over 65 years.

Causes
➤ Increased uric acid intake, e.g. high purine diet or production, e.g. myelo/lymphoproliferative disorders.
➤ Reduced uric acid excretion, e.g. alcohol, drugs such as thiazide diuretics, renal failure.

Diagnosis
➤ History.
➤ Examination – the first metatarsalphalangeal joint is affected in 90% of cases.
➤ Elevated serum uric acid (although may be normal).
➤ Synovial fluid aspirate – negatively birefringent needle-shaped crystals under polarised light.

Management[4]
➤ Address modifiable predisposing factors.
➤ NSAIDs (with caution).
➤ Colchicine if NSAIDs contraindicated.
➤ Steroids (orally, intramuscularly or by intra-articular injection) if NSAIDs/colchicine contraindicated or ineffective.
➤ Consider long-term treatment with a xanthine-oxidase inhibitor, e.g. allopurinol

if more than one attack per year, chronic tophaceous disease or renal failure.

➤ In patients intolerant of, or resistant to, allopurinol, uricosuric drugs such as sulfinpyrazone or probenecid could be prescribed (NICE has recently recommended febuxostat [a non-purine xanthine-oxidase inhibitor] as an alternative to these).[5]

Pseudogout

➤ An inflammatory joint condition caused by deposition of calcium pyrophosphate crystals.
➤ More common in older people.
➤ Predisposing factors include:
  — dehydration
  — intercurrent illness.
➤ Episodes are characterised by an acute mono- or oligoarticular arthritis.
➤ The knee is most frequently affected.
➤ Positively birefringent crystals are seen on synovial fluid analysis.
➤ X-rays may show chondrocalcinosis.
➤ Treatment options include:
  — simple analgesia (caution with NSAIDs)
  — aspiration (may help relieve symptoms)
  — oral or intra-articular steroids
  — colchicine.

POLYMYALGIA RHEUMATICA

➤ An inflammatory syndrome characterised by pain and stiffness in the neck, shoulders and pelvic girdle.
➤ Peak incidence 70–80 years of age.
➤ More prevalent in women.
➤ More common in Caucasians.
➤ Diagnosis is based upon history, clinical examination findings, raised ESR and response to steroids.
➤ Start prednisolone at a dose of 10–15 mg daily tapering the dose according to ESR and symptoms.
➤ Most patients require low dose maintenance steroids for at least 6–12 months.

REFERENCES

1 National Institute for Health and Clinical Excellence. *The Care and Management of Osteoarthritis in Adults. NICE clinical guideline 59.* London: NIHCE; 2008. Available at: www.nice.org.uk/cg59 (accessed 26 May 2010).
2 National Institute for Health and Clinical Excellence. *The Management of Rheumatoid Arthritis in Adults. NICE clinical guideline 79.* London: NIHCE; 2009. Available at: www.nice.org.uk/cg79 (accessed 26 May 2010).
3 National Rheumatoid Arthritis Society. www.nras.org.uk
4 Jordan KM *et al.* British Society for Rheumatology and British Health Professionals in Rheumatology guideline for the management of Gout. *Rheumatology.* 2007; **46**: 1372–4.
5 National Institute for Health and Clinical Excellence. *Febuxostat for the Management of Hyperuricaemia in People with Gout: final appraisal determination.* London: NIHCE; 2008. Available at: www.nice.org.uk/TA164 (accessed 26 May 2010).

CHAPTER 17

Mental health problems

GENERAL
➤ Common in the older population.
➤ Important conditions include:
  — dementia
  — delirium
  — depression
  — anxiety
  — sleep disturbance
  — chronic schizophrenia.

NATIONAL SERVICE FRAMEWORK FOR OLDER PEOPLE: STANDARD 7: MENTAL HEALTH (2001)[1]
Aims
➤ To promote good mental health in older people.
➤ To ensure early diagnosis.
➤ To provide access to specialist care and an integrated approach to assessment and treatment.
➤ To support carers.

DEMENTIA
Definition
➤ Dementia is a term used to describe a group of illnesses in which there is progressive impairment of memory and other cognitive function.

Main types of dementia in the older population
➤ Alzheimer's disease (60% of cases).
➤ Vascular dementia (20% of cases).
➤ Dementia with Lewy bodies (15% of cases).
➤ Other causes include frontotemporal and subcortical types.

Statistics
➤ 700 000 people in UK have dementia.
➤ Prevalence increases with age:
  — 5% of >65s.
  — 20% of >80s.
➤ Estimated number of cases by 2026: 840 000; by 2050: 1.2 million.
➤ Annual cost of dementia care is estimated to be £17 billion.

Clinical features
➤ Cognitive function:
  — progressive loss of short term memory
  — difficulty in registration and recall of new information
  — language problems, e.g. repetition.
➤ Behavioural changes:
  — aggression, disinhibition, social withdrawal, wandering, disorientation
  — inability to perform usual activities of daily living.
➤ Psychiatric problems:
  — associated mood disorder
  — delusions/hallucinations.
➤ Physical debility:
  — self-neglect
  — incontinence
  — falls.

Diagnosis
Collateral history
➤ Patient's account may be unreliable.
➤ Background information from relatives, friends, neighbours and health professionals can be invaluable.
➤ Assists with diagnosis.
➤ Highlights problems that may be encountered on a day-to-day basis, e.g. difficulties with personal care, domestic tasks, self-administration of medication, attendance at medical appointments, use of public transport and financial issues.

Assessment of cognitive function (see Chapter 8)
➤ Abbreviated Mental Test Score (AMTS).
➤ Mini Mental State Examination (MMSE).
➤ Used in conjunction with other methods of assessment, these tests can assist in the diagnosis.
➤ *MMSE*   *Degree of cognitive impairment*
   22–6   Mild
   10–21 Moderate
    0–9   Severe

Clinical examination
➤ May illicit clues to diagnosis, e.g. self-neglect.
➤ Important to exclude other pathology as a cause for symptoms.

Baseline investigations
➤ Blood tests (full blood count, renal/liver/thyroid function tests, calcium, vitamin B12, folate ± syphilis serology).
➤ CT/MRI brain.

Management
Non-pharmacological
➤ Psychological interventions include cognitive, behavioural and emotion-focused approaches.
➤ Assistance with activities of daily living.
➤ Reduction of carer burden through education and support.

Pharmacological

➤ Patients exhibiting extreme behavioural problems may require small doses of sedative medication, e.g. haloperidol, lorazepam.
➤ Cholinesterase inhibitors are licensed for use in mild/moderate Alzheimer's disease (AD).
➤ Memantine (NMDA antagonist) can be used in more severe cases of AD.

Memory clinics

➤ Provide a multidisciplinary specialist service.
➤ May be run by psychogeriatricians, consultants in care of the old or neurologists.
➤ Aims are to assess and treat cognitive and behavioural symptoms, monitor response to therapy, slow progression of disease and provide information/support to carers.
➤ National Service Framework suggests that patients should be referred for specialist advice early and particularly in certain instances:
— uncertain diagnosis
— difficult behavioural or psychological symptoms
— safety concerns
— risk of abuse or self-harm
— determination of mental capacity.

Carers

➤ Family members, friends or neighbours often take on role of informal carer when an older person develops dementia.
➤ Pressures may be emotional, social, financial and physical.
➤ Respite should be offered in the form of day centre care, sitter services and either short- or long-term admission to a convalescence facility or psychogeriatric ward.
➤ Charitable organisations such as the Alzheimer's Disease Society can provide information and support for carers.

Alzheimer's disease

➤ Commonest form of dementia in the older population.
➤ Affects 15 million people worldwide.
➤ A neurodegenerative disease associated with characteristic pathological changes in neocortex and hippocampus:
— neurofibrillary tangles (containing tau protein)
— senile plaques (with extracellular deposits of β-amyloid)
— loss of neurones and neuronal synapses (including loss of cholinergic transmission).
➤ Aetiology remains unknown.

Clinical Features (Diagnostic and Statistical Manual of Mental Disorders)[2]

a   Development of multiple cognitive deficits manifested by both:
   1   Memory impairment (impaired ability to learn new information or to recall previously learned information).
   2   One (or more) of the following cognitive disturbances:
     • aphasia (language disturbance)
     • apraxia (impaired ability to carry out motor activities despite intact motor function)

- agnosia (failure to recognise or identify objects despite intact sensory function)
- disturbance in executive functioning (planning, organisation).

b Cognitive deficits in A1 and A2 each cause significant impairment in social or occupational functioning and represent a significant decline from a previous level of functioning.

c Course characterised by gradual onset and continuing cognitive decline.

d Cognitive deficits in A1 and A2 are not due to any of the following:
  — other central nervous conditions that cause progressive deficits in memory and cognition (e.g. cerebrovascular disease, Parkinson's disease, Huntington's chorea, subdural haematoma, normal pressure hydrocephalus, tumour)
  — systemic conditions that are known to cause dementia (e.g. hypothyroidism, deficiencies in vitamin B12/folate/niacin, hypercalcaemia, neurosyphilis and HIV)
  — substance-induced conditions.

e Deficits do not occur exclusively during the course of the delirium.

f Disturbance is not better accounted for by another disorder, e.g. depression.

Drug therapy in Alzheimer's disease
CHOLINESTERASE INHIBITORS

➤ Alzheimer's disease is characterised by a cholinergic deficit.
➤ Cholinesterase inhibitors enhance cholinergic neurotransmission by delaying breakdown of acetylcholine.
➤ Three drugs (donepezil, galantamine and rivastigmine) are licensed in UK for use in mild/moderate AD.
➤ Patients should be on highest tolerable dose for maximal effect.
➤ It may be worthwhile switching to a different agent when first begins to lose effect.
➤ Side-effects include gastrointestinal upset, headache, dizziness, fatigue, syncope and bradycardias.
➤ Current UK prescribing distribution:
  — donepezil   70%
  — galantamine   18%
  — rivastigmine   12%
➤ Drug costs approximately £42 million/year (may be offset by delay in admissions to residential/nursing care facilities).

MEMANTINE

➤ Excessive activation of the NMDA (N-methyl-D-aspartate) receptor by glutamate (an excitatory amino acid) may contribute to destruction of cholinergic neurones.
➤ Memantine is an NMDA receptor antagonist.
➤ Licensed for use in moderate/severe AD in UK since 2002.
➤ May stabilise symptoms.
➤ Optimum dose 20 mg/day.
➤ Potential side-effects include confusion, hallucinations, dizziness, headaches and fatigue.
➤ Trials under way to assess efficacy in other dementia types.

NICE Guidance on drug prescription (2007)[3]

➤ Donepezil, galantamine and rivastigmine are recommended for the treatment of patients with moderately severe AD only.
➤ MMSE score must be between 10 and 20 (other markers of severity can be used should the MMSE be considered unreliable).

➤ Cognition, global/behavioural functioning and activities of daily living must be assessed before prescription.
➤ Compliance must be assured.
➤ Drug should only be continued if, at 2–4 months, specialist assessment shows improvement or no deterioration in MMSE score, or there is evidence of improvement based on behavioural or functional assessment.
➤ Patients should be reviewed every 6 months and treatment only continued while MMSE remains at or above 10 and their global, functional and behavioural condition remains at a level where the drug is considered to be having a worthwhile effect.
➤ Carers' views on the patient's condition should be sought at each assessment.
➤ Memantine is not recommended as a treatment except as part of a clinical study.

Vascular dementia
➤ Second most common form of dementia.
➤ Characterised by abrupt onset and step-wise deterioration.
➤ Certain abilities may remain unaffected depending on areas of brain involved.
➤ Risk factors include:
  — stroke
  — transient ischaemic attacks
  — atrial fibrillation
  — hypertension
  — diabetes mellitus
  — smoking
  — hypercholesterolaemia
  — family history of vascular disease.
➤ CT/MRI brain will show evidence of ischaemic damage.
➤ Primary prevention is important in high-risk groups.
➤ Secondary prevention is paramount in reducing chance of further events.

Dementia with Lewy bodies
➤ Microscopic deposits (Lewy bodies) cause damage to nerve cells.
➤ Characterised by parkinsonism, visual hallucinations and falls in addition to progressive cognitive impairment.

NICE and the Social Care Institute for Excellence (2006)[4]
➤ Current priorities:
  — people with dementia should not be excluded from services because of their diagnosis
  — valid consent should be obtained – if a person lacks capacity to make a decision, the provisions of the Mental Health Act 2005[5] should be followed
  — coordination and integration of health and social services is vital
  — memory assessment services should be the single point of referral for all people with a possible diagnosis of dementia
  — structural brain imaging (MRI or CT brain) should be used to establish the diagnosis
  — the needs of carers' should be identified and met
  — challenging behaviour should be comprehensively assessed and individual care plans developed
  — staff working with older people with dementia should be appropriately trained
  — acute hospitals should be able to meet the needs of people with dementia.

National Dementia Strategy UK (2009)[6]
➤ A 5-year plan with 17 objectives focusing on three key areas:
  — raising awareness
  — making an early diagnosis
  — improving quality of care.
➤ Objectives:
  — to raise public and professional awareness and understanding
  — to provide good-quality early diagnosis, support and treatment
  — to make good-quality information available for patients and their carers
  — to enable easy access to care, support and advice following diagnosis
  — to develop structured peer support and learning networks
  — to improve community personal support services
  — to ensure carers' needs are recognised and met
  — to improve the quality of care for people with dementia in general
    hospitals
  — to improve intermediate care for people with dementia
  — to consider how housing support, housing-related services, technology and
    telecare can provide support to patients and their carers
  — to improve the quality of care for people with dementia in care homes
  — to improve end of life care
  — to ensure that professionals working with people with dementia are
    appropriately trained
  — to coordinate joint commissioning of health and social services
  — to improve assessment and regulation of health and care services
  — to provide information about dementia research
  — to provide national and regional support for local services to enable
    implementation of the strategy.

DELIRIUM
Definition
➤ A syndrome characterised by concurrent disturbance of consciousness and
  attention, perception, thinking, memory, psychomotor behaviour, emotion and
  the sleep-wake cycle (ICD-10: International Classification of Disease).[7]

Statistics
➤ Up to 30% of medical inpatients are affected.
➤ Increases morbidity and mortality rates, length of hospital stay and rate of
  institutionalisation.

Predisposing factors
➤ Old age.
➤ Dementia.
➤ Past history of delirium.
➤ Significant comorbidities.
➤ Sensory impairment (vision/hearing).
➤ Change of environment (often in association with pre-existing dementia).

Causes
➤ Infection, e.g. urine, chest.
➤ Drugs, e.g. antibiotics, anticholinergics, anticonvulsants, anti-Parkinsonian drugs,
  opiate analgesics, psychotropics, steroids.
➤ Drug withdrawal, e.g. alcohol, benzodiazepines.

➤ Metabolic, e.g. electrolyte disturbances, dehydration, hepatic dysfunction, hyper/
hypoglycaemia, hyper/hypothyroidism, hypoxia.
➤ Neurological, e.g. stroke, transient ischaemic attacks, postictal, space-occupying
lesions, meningitis, encephalitis.

Clinical features

➤ Acute onset (hours/days).
➤ Fluctuating intensity.
➤ Impaired consciousness.
➤ Disorientation in time, place and person.
➤ Poor attention.
➤ Visual hallucinations.
➤ Some patients become withdrawn ('quiet delirium').
➤ Most recover within 4 weeks but symptoms may last 6 months.

Complications

➤ Falls and subsequent injury.
➤ Consequences of medication non-compliance.
➤ Loss of functional independence.
➤ Incontinence.
➤ Inadequate nutrition.
➤ Dehydration.
➤ Over-sedation.
➤ Pressure sores in hypoactive cases.

Assessment

➤ Investigations to consider include routine blood tests, urinalysis and brain CT.
➤ Diagnostic scale, e.g. CAM – Confusion Assessment Method (1990):[8]
  — feature 1: acute onset and fluctuating course
  — feature 2: inattention
  — feature 3: disorganised thinking
  — feature 4: altered level of consciousness.
➤ Diagnosis by the Confusion Assessment Method requires presence of features 1
and 2 and either feature 3 or 4.

Management

➤ Identify high risk individuals.
➤ Treat reversible causes.
➤ Additional steps:

Non-drug strategies

➤ Nurse in a safe area, preferably a side room, with adequate lighting and low noise
levels.
➤ Avoid inter/intra-ward transfers.
➤ Maintain continuity of nursing staff if possible and keep number of staff to a
minimum.
➤ Reassure and talk calmly.
➤ Ensure provision of glasses and hearing aids.
➤ Provide familiar objects and clocks to assist orientation.
➤ Explain situation to visitors and encourage their support.
➤ Avoid physical restraints.

Medication
➤ Sedation may need to be considered in some cases:
— risk of self-harm or injury to others
— severe agitation
— essential investigations or treatment required.
➤ Low doses of antipsychotics (e.g. haloperidol) or benzodiazepines (e.g. lorazepam) can be used.

DEPRESSION
Statistics
➤ Most common psychiatric disorder in those over 65 years (affects 10–15%).
➤ 3–5% over 65 years have severe depression.
➤ Associated with high suicide rate.
➤ Increases morbidity and mortality.

Precipitating factors
➤ Bereavement.
➤ Retirement.
➤ Change in living circumstances, e.g. institutionalisation.
➤ Poor health (twice as many people with chronic illnesses have depression compared to the physically well).
➤ Disability.
➤ Social isolation.
➤ Past history of depression.
➤ Family history of mood disorder.
➤ Certain drugs, e.g. β-blockers, neuroleptics, steroids, opiates and alcohol.

Clinical features
➤ Low mood.
➤ Anhedonia.
➤ Sleep disturbance (early morning wakening).
➤ Fatigue.
➤ Poor memory and concentration.
➤ Agitation.
➤ Feelings of guilt, helplessness or hopelessness.
➤ Loss of appetite and weight.
➤ Preoccupation with death.
➤ Suicidal thoughts.
➤ Delusions.
➤ Somatic symptoms with no identifiable physical cause.

Risk factors for suicide
➤ Male.
➤ Previous suicidal attempt.
➤ Bereavement.
➤ Painful medical conditions.
➤ Social isolation.
➤ Alcohol dependence.

Diagnosis
➤ May be difficult to diagnose in older people:
— patients may minimise their feelings of sadness

   — presentation with physical complaints is common

   — concomitant illness may challenge assessment.

➤ Geriatric Depression Scale[9] assesses mainly cognitive aspects rather than physical symptoms:

➤ *Scores*

   — 5–8   mild

   — 8–11   moderate

   — 12–15 severe

➤ Assess suicide risk.

➤ Identify any precipitants.

➤ Exclude physical causes of low mood, e.g. hypothyroidism.

➤ Differential diagnoses include anxiety, grief and dementia.

Management
Psychological therapies

➤ Cognitive behavioural therapy, interpersonal therapy or brief, focused analytical therapy have been shown to be effective.

Social

➤ Address social isolation.

Antidepressant drugs

➤ Augment noradrenergic and/or serotoninergic transmission.

➤ Treatment duration generally 6 months to 2 years (longer if recurrent episodes).

➤ Established antidepressants include tricyclics and monoamino oxidase inhibitors – these have been largely superseded by new therapies.

➤ New treatments include:

   — SSRIs (Selective Serotonin Reuptake Inhibitors), e.g. citalopram, fluoxetine, paroxetine and sertraline

   — SNRIs (Serotonin/Noradrenaline Reuptake Inhibitors), e.g. venlafaxine

   — NaSSAs (Noradrenaline and Specific Serotoninergic Antidepressants), e.g. mirtazepine.

➤ Advantages of newer antidepressants:

   — better tolerated

   — less cardiotoxic

   — less lethal in overdose.

➤ Lithium augmentation may be considered in poorly responsive cases.

Electroconvulsive therapy

➤ In severe cases unresponsive to other treatment methods.

National Service Framework suggests specialist psychiatric review in certain situations

➤ Unclear diagnosis.

➤ Complex symptoms, e.g. multiple physical problems.

➤ Suicide risk.

➤ Inadequate response to first-line treatment.

➤ Psychotic symptoms, e.g. delusions.

ANXIETY

➤ Generalised anxiety disorder is characterised by frequent, persistent worry and anxiety for at least 6 months.

➤ More common in women.
➤ May be a new diagnosis in later life in association with other psychiatric problems such as depression, physical illness or as a side-effect of medication.
➤ Symptoms include:
  — poor concentration
  — irritability
  — sleep disturbance
  — fatigue
  — palpitations
  — nausea
  — shortness of breath
  — sweating
  — urinary frequency
  — headaches
  — dizziness.

NICE Treatment Guidance (2004)[10]

➤ Benzodiazepines should not usually be used for more than 2–4 weeks.
➤ Long-term management options include:
  — cognitive behavioural therapy (CBT)
  — selective serotonin reuptake inhibitors
  — self-help based on CBT principles.
➤ If one type of intervention does not work an alternative should be offered.
➤ If symptoms have not resolved following two interventions, referral to specialist mental health services should be considered.

SLEEP DISORDERS
Definition

➤ Sleep disturbance is defined as any disruptive pattern of sleep such as problems falling asleep, staying asleep, excessive sleep or abnormal behaviours associated with sleep.

Statistics

➤ Sleep disturbance common in older people.
➤ 12–25% of healthy older people report chronic insomnia.
➤ Higher rates seen in those with physical or psychiatric illness.
➤ Tends to be underdiagnosed (sufferers may incorrectly believe it is part of normal ageing) and undertreated.

Normal sleep pattern

➤ NREM (non-rapid eye movement): four stages (deepest sleep in stages 3 and 4).
➤ REM (rapid eye movement): dream sleep.

Factors predisposing to sleep disturbance

➤ Lifestyle changes, e.g. daytime inactivity with intermittent sleep episodes can lead to less fatigue at night (irregular sleeping schedule).
➤ Behavioural practices, e.g. association of bedtime with other activities such as reading, watching television.
➤ Psychiatric disorders, e.g. anxiety, depression, dementia, delirium.
➤ Physical illness, for example:
  — pain (arthritis, angina, gastro-oesophageal reflux, calf ischaemia, cramps)
  — urinary symptoms (incontinence, nocturia)

➤ — respiratory symptoms (congestive cardiac failure, chronic obstructive airways disease, sleep apnoea)
— other (restless legs syndrome).
➤ Drugs, e.g. caffeine, alcohol, nicotine, antidepressants, antihypertensives.

Sleep history
➤ Identify predisposing factors.
➤ Establish quality, duration and timing of sleep.

Effects of sleep deprivation
➤ Fatigue.
➤ Poor concentration.
➤ Increased tendency to fall.
➤ More likely to make errors, e.g. leaving gas/electrical appliances on.

Management
Non-pharmacological
➤ General advice:
— relieve contributing medical/psychiatric symptoms where possible
— establish regular bed/awakening times
— avoid daytime naps
— use sleep-promotion interventions, e.g. ensure quiet environment, warm drink before bed, avoid other activities while in bed.
➤ Cognitive behavioural therapy.
➤ Exercise (selected patients).

Pharmacological
➤ Consider low dose sedatives in resistant cases for short periods only, e.g. 3–4 weeks.
➤ Side-effects of benzodiazepines, e.g. temazepam include tolerance, addiction and daytime sleepiness (increases risk of falls).

CHRONIC SCHIZOPHRENIA
Definition
➤ Chronic schizophrenia is defined as a condition characterised by disorders of thought, perception, memory and personality.

Statistics
➤ Majority of cases present in adolescence or early adulthood.
➤ Prevalence is 0.1–0.5% in over-65s.
➤ Cases in later life may be due to new onset disease or life-long illness.
➤ 5–10% of older people have psychotic episodes – most associated with dementia; 20% due to schizophrenia.

Associations in late-onset schizophrenia
➤ Female gender.
➤ Social isolation.
➤ Sensory impairment (deafness/poor vision).
➤ Premorbid paranoid personality traits.
➤ Not associated with family history or obstetric complications as in younger onset cases.

Clinical features
➤ Positive symptoms:
  — delusions
  — hallucinations
  — disorganised thinking and speech.
➤ Negative symptoms:
  — social withdrawal
  — low motivation
  — self-neglect
  — often absent in older people.

Diagnosis
➤ Schneider's First Rank Symptoms[11] (characteristic/diagnostic features)
  — auditory hallucinations (third person, running commentary)
  — thought disorder (withdrawal, insertion, broadcasting)
  — passivity experiences (delusions of control)
  — delusional perception.
➤ Physical causes should be excluded.
➤ Differential diagnoses include:
  — dementia
  — delirium
  — depression
  — paranoid personality.

Management
Non-drug strategies
➤ Social interaction.
➤ Cognitive behavioural therapy.

Drug therapy
➤ Atypical antipsychotic drugs treatment of choice.
➤ Olanzepine, quetiapine and risperidone commonly prescribed.
➤ These lack troublesome side-effects of typical antipsychotics such as chlorpromazine (parkinsonism, tardive dyskinesia).
➤ 'Start low, go slow' approach should be adopted with reference to dose and up-titrations.
➤ Assistance of carers or district nurses may be required to ensure medication compliance (risperidone can be given in a long-acting intramuscular form otherwise).
➤ Approximately 50% of patients respond to treatment.

REFERENCES
1 Department of Health. *National Service Framework for Older People*. London: Department of Health; 2001. Available at: www.dh.gov.uk/en/publicationsandstatistics/publications/publicationspolicyandguidance/dh_4003066 (accessed 26 May 2010).
2 American Psychiatric Association. *Diagnostic and Statistical Manual of Mental Disorders*. 4th ed. (text revision). Washington, DC: American Psychiatric Association; 2000.
3 National Institute for Health and Clinical Excellence. *Donepezil, galantamine, rivastigmine (review) and memantine for the Treatment of Alzheimer's Disease (amended). NICE technology appraisal guidance 111*. London: NIHCE; 2007. Available at: www.nice.org.uk/nicemedia/pdf/ta111qrgsept07.pdf (accessed 26 May 2010).
4 National Institute for Health and Clinical Excellence and Social Care Institute for Excellence.

Dementia: supporting people with dementia and their carers in health and social care. NICE clinical guideline 42. London: NIHCE; 2006. Available at: www.nice.org.uk/cg42 (accessed 26 May 2010).

5 Office of the Public Guardian. *Mental Capacity Act 2005*. Birmingham: Office of the Public Guardian; 2005. Available at: www.publicguardian.gov.uk/mca/mca.htm (accessed 26 May 2010).

6 Department of Health. *Living Well with Dementia: a national dementia strategy*. London: Department of Health; 2009. Available at: www.dh.gov.uk/en/publicationsandstatistics/publications/publicationspolicyandguidance/dh_094058 (accessed 26 May 2010).

7 World Health Organization. *International Statistical Classification of Diseases and Related Health Problems*. Geneva: WHO; 1992.

8 Inouye SK *et al.* Clarifying confusion: the confusion assessment method. A new method for detection of delirium. *Ann Intern Med*. 1990; **113**: 941–8.

9 Yesavage *et al.* Development and validation of a geriatric depression screening scale: a preliminary report. *J Psychiatr Res*. 1983; **17**: 37–49.

10 National Institute for Health and Clinical Excellence. *Anxiety: management of anxiety (panic disorder, with or without agoraphobia, and generalized anxiety disorder) in adults in primary, secondary and community care. NICE clinical guideline 22*. London: NIHCE; 2004. Available at: www.nice.org.uk/cg22 (accessed 26 May 2010).

11 Schneider K. *Clinical Psychopathology*. New York: Grune and Stratton; 1959.

FURTHER READING

National Institute for Health and Clinical Excellence. *Depression: the treatment and management of depression in adults. NICE clinical guideline 90*. London: NIHCE; 2009. www.nice.org.uk/cg90

Royal College of Physicians. *Concise guidance to good practice: the Prevention, diagnosis and management of delirium in older people. National guidelines 6*. London: RCP; 2006. www.rcplondon.ac.uk/pubs/books/pdmd/DeliriumConciseGuide.pdf

CHAPTER 18

Alcohol and drug abuse

Rhodri Edwards

ALCOHOL

➤ The word 'alcohol' is derived from the Arabic *al-kuhl* literally meaning 'the kohl' (antimony powder used to brighten the eyes).

Recommended daily alcohol consumption

➤ Current UK government recommendations: women 2–3 units of alcohol per day and adult men 3–4 units per day.
➤ National Institute on Alcohol Abuse and Alcoholism in the USA recommends people over 65 should consume no more than 1 standard drink per day, 7 standard drinks per week.

Alcohol units and conversion

➤ One unit of alcohol is equal to approximately 8 g of absolute alcohol per 10 mL, as found in:
 — half a pint (285 mL) of normal strength (3.5%) beer
 — a glass of wine (9%) (125 mL)
 — a small glass of sherry (50 mL)
➤ 'single of spirits' (25 mL).

Statistics

➤ 15% of women and 22% of men aged ≥65 years report consume more alcohol than recommended (General Household Survey, 2007).
➤ 3% of women and 8% of men aged ≥65 years are heavy alcohol users (General Household Survey, 2007).
➤ The prevalence of mild alcohol dependence in people aged 65–9 is 17 per 1 000 and decreases to 9 per 1 000 in people aged 70–4.
➤ 30% of hospitalised older people on general medical wards may be heavy alcohol users.
➤ 50% of older psychiatric in patients are heavy users of alcohol.
➤ In men >40 years and post-menopausal women, modest alcohol consumption (1–2 units/day) has a protective affect against coronary artery disease and stroke.

Classification of older alcohol misuse

Early onset	Two thirds of older alcohol misusers. Lifelong pattern of problems with alcohol. Develop alcohol problems in 20–30s. Higher proportion of men, lower socio-economic status, strong family history of alcohol problems. More likely to have psychiatric illness, alcohol-related chronic illness (e.g. cirrhosis) and cognitive loss may be more severe and less reversible. Less compliant with treatment programmes.
Late onset	One third of older alcohol misusers. Develop alcohol problems in their 40–50s. Higher proportion of women, higher socio-economic class and level of education. May be triggered or exacerbated by a major life event. Fewer physical and mental health problems. Better prognosis and compliance with treatment.

Risk factors for alcohol-related problems
Demographic
➤ *Age*: rates of alcohol abuse and dependence are lower among older adults. This may be because:
  — heavy drinkers die earlier
  — increasing medical problems and comorbidity make drinking undesirable or hazardous
  — biological changes (such as decreased body water:fat ratio, decreased hepatic blood flow, inefficient liver enzymes, renal impairment) reduce the amount of alcohol older people are able to consume
  — cultural factors such as prohibition affect the attitude of older people to alcohol
  — inaccurate methods of measuring drinking in older adults.
➤ *Gender*: males are at a greater risk than females
➤ *Socio-economic group*:
  — higher socio-economic groups are more likely to consume alcohol and drink smaller amounts more frequently
  — higher socio-economic class is associated with higher rates of alcohol consumption and dependence
  — lower socio-economic groups have a higher proportion of people who abstain from alcohol as well as people who are heavy consumers of alcohol and require hospital admission with problems such as alcohol psychosis, acute intoxication and liver cirrhosis.
➤ *Living arrangements and partnerships*: co-habiting, being single, divorced or separated are associated with increased risk of hazardous drinking. However, among older people, married women show significant levels of alcohol consumption.
➤ *Ethnic group*:
  — the Caucasian population generally consume more alcohol and are at most risk of alcohol related problems
  — average alcohol consumption is generally lower in the Afro-Caribbean population and communities originating from South Asia although they maybe disproportionately affected by the adverse consequences of alcohol consumption
  — people of Pakistani or Bangladeshi origin are least likely to have consumed alcohol in the previous week (~5%) compared with white British/white other (~68%)
  — heavy consumption of alcohol (particularly spirits) is more common in Sikh men
  — people from Ireland may also be of increased risk.

Familial and genetic

➤ *Family history*: up to 50% of heavy alcohol users have a family history of alcohol misuse. A history of alcoholism in a first degree relative is the most powerful predictor of alcohol misuse.
➤ *Genetic factors*: twin studies showed greater concordance of alcoholism in monozygotic twins. Dizygotic twins also show increased risk ratios. However, 40–70% of co-twins of alcoholics do not have alcohol-related problems. Genes, therefore, probably have a predisposing role interacting with other environmental factors.

Medical and social problems

➤ *Medical problems*: chronic illness, chronic pain, physical disability, insomnia.
➤ *Psychiatric illness*: schizophrenia, bipolar disorders, major depression, social phobia, panic disorder, post traumatic stress, attention deficit hyperactivity disorder, antisocial and borderline personality disorder.
➤ *Personality type*: conduct disorder and antisocial behaviour are strong predictors.
➤ *Emotional and social problems*: major life events (bereavement, divorce, loss of employment), financial difficulty, isolation, social exclusion, low self-esteem, impaired self-care, reduced coping skills.

Society

➤ *Availability and pricing*:
  — alcohol is cheap in relation to cost of living indices and the real price of alcohol has declined steadily over the last 50 years.
➤ *Culture and customs*: the prevailing attitude of society and the community probably influences the consumption of alcohol. Different cultures use alcohol in many different ways such as an important component of a meal, for leisure time or simply for intoxicating effect. Other cultures on the whole abstain from alcohol.

Screening
CAGE Questions

C – Ever decided to cut down?
A – Do you get annoyed when people talk about how much you drink?
G – Do you have guilt feelings about your drinking?
E – Do you ever need an eye opener to get going the next day?

Sensitivity drops with age, however, specificity is maintained.

MAST-G: Michigan Alcohol Screening Test – Geriatric Version

This questionnaire asks 24 questions. Scoring 5 or more 'yes' response's is indicative of alcohol problems. It is more sensitive and specific for older people. A shortened version is also available.

Laboratory investigations

➤ The role of blood test in the diagnosis of alcohol misuse is limited. They may, however, raise suspicion of an alcohol-related problem. The γ-glutamyl transferase (γ-GT) and mean corpuscular volume (MCV) have been widely used as potential markers. A man with a MCV >98 fL and γ-GT >50 iu/L has a 62% chance of admitting to drinking over 450 g of alcohol per week.
➤ Other laboratory findings include low platelets, reduced urea, raised aspartate transaminase and alanine aminotransferase, elevated fasting triglycerides and

raised alcohol concentration in breath and urine (A blood alcohol level of 80 mg/100 mL is the legal limit for driving in the UK. A breath test result of 35 μg/100 mL is equivalent to a blood alcohol level of 80 mg/100 mL).

Alcohol and health problems

Alcohol use can cause a wide range of physical, psychological and social problems.

TABLE 18.1 Alcohol related health problems with associated clinical features/ clinical consequences

Health problem	Clinical consequences/clinical features
Malnutrition and vitamin deficiencies	Deficiencies in vitamin B_1 (thiamine), A, D, B_6, E and folate.
Liver disease	Fatty liver, acute hepatitis, cirrhosis of the liver.
Gastrointestinal disease	Oesophagitis, gastritis, pancreatitis, diarrhoea.
Malignancy	Carcinoma of the mouth, larynx, oesophagus, pancreas, colon and liver.
Neurological	Strokes, cerebral atrophy, subdural haematoma, dementia, peripheral neuropathy.
Wernicke's encephalopathy	Characterized by oculomotor disturbances (nystagmus, gaze palsy, opthalmoplegia), cerebellar ataxia and mental confusion (disorientation, inattention, poor responsiveness). Stupor and coma may develop. Caused by thiamine deficiency.
Korsakoff's syndrome	Characterised by various degrees of anterograde and reterograde amnesia with relative preservation of other intellectual functions. Potentially reversible with early treatment with thiamine but often recovery is incomplete.
Alcohol dementia	Cognitive deficits caused by cortical atrophy from alcohol abuse.
Psychological	Alcohol induced anxiety disorders, hallucinations, amnesia, alcohol psychosis, sleep disorders, overdose, suicide.
Cardiovascular	Arrhythmias, cardiomyopathy, hypertension.
Musculoskeletal	Acute and chronic myopathy, osteoporosis.
Blood	Anaemia (direct effect on erythropoiesis, folate deficiency, derangement of iron metabolism, haemolysis), neutropenia and impairment of leucocyte function, thrombocytopenia.
Endocrine	Hypogonadism (loss of libido, testicular atrophy), gynaecomastia, loss of body hair, pseudo-Cushing's syndrome.
Metabolic	Hypoglycaemia, ketoacidosis, disorders of fat and uric acid metabolism.
Drug interactions	Multiple drug interactions occur with serious potential consequences.
Accidental injury	Falls, fractures, traumatic injury, motor vehicle accidents.

Specific considerations for alcohol in older people

➤ Older people are less likely to disclose information about drinking and are likely to underreport alcohol consumption. In one study, which specifically asked older people about adding alcohol to tea or coffee, the number of heavy drinkers doubled from those who admitted to drinking alcohol on its own.

➤ Health professionals are reluctant to ask about alcohol use.
➤ Misconceptions exist that alcohol is not a significant problem in the older population.
➤ Biomedical presentation of alcohol abuse is common and often underrecognised, i.e falls, confusion, dehydration, malnutrition, myopathy, incontinence and traumatic injury.
➤ Screening instruments have not been designed to be used with older people.
➤ Withdrawal symptoms may be more severe and longer lasting in older people and may occur after less frequent or less heavy alcohol use.

Management and treatment

➤ *Assessment*: recognition of alcohol problems and engaging the patient are vital first steps.
➤ *Brief intervention*: one or more counselling sessions including assessment, motivational work, patient education and feedback, contracting (keeping a drink diary and setting goals and incentives to reduce consumption) and use support materials.
➤ *Specialist treatments*: community alcohol teams, inpatient detoxification units, structured day centre or residential programmes. Alcoholics Anonymous offer support. Further counselling, group therapy or cognitive behavioural therapy programmes may be helpful.

Detoxification

➤ Inpatient detoxification is likely to be appropriate for frail, vulnerable older people with significant comorbidity.
➤ Benzodiazepines: chlordiazepoxide: typical regimen 20–30 mg chlordiazepoxide four times daily reducing to zero over 5 days. Dose adjustment for frail and older people is appropriate.
➤ Vitamin therapy: parentral thiamine to prevent Wernicke-Korsakoff syndrome.

Drugs to maintain abstinence

➤ Disulfiram: prevent breakdown of alcohol by acetaldehyde dehydrogenase causing unpleasant reaction (flushing, headache, palpitations, nausea and vomiting) if taken with alcohol. Cardiovascular toxicity and can precipitate acute confusional state. A number of studies recommend disulfiram is *not* used in the old.
➤ Acamprosate: γ-aminobutyric acid analogue can be used as an adjunct to psychological therapy.
➤ Naltrexone is an opioid antagonist and is not licensed in UK to treat alcohol dependence.

TOBACCO AND NICOTINE DEPENDENCE
Statistics

➤ 13% of men and 13% of women aged ≥60 reported smoking cigarettes (General Household Survey, 2007).
➤ 49% of men and 29% of women aged ≥60 reported previous regular cigarette smoking (General Household Survey, 2007).
➤ Prevalence of smoking decreases with age.
➤ Married people are less likely to smoke.
➤ Smoking is related with significant morbidity and mortality including coronary artery disease, Stroke, peripheral vascular disease, abdominal aortic aneurysm, chronic obstructive pulmonary disease (COPD), pneumonia and multiple

neoplastic diseases – acute myeloid leukaemia, bladder, esophageal, laryngeal, lung, oral, throat, cervical, kidney, stomach and pancreatic cancers.

Benefits of stopping smoking
➤ Substantial immediate and long-term benefits.
➤ After 3–9 months, breathing problems improve and lung function increases by up to 10%.
➤ After 1 year, risk of myocardial infarction (MI) falls to 50% of that of a smoker.
➤ After 10 years, risk of lung cancer falls to 30–50% of that of a smoker.
➤ After 15 years, risk of heart attack falls to same level as someone who has never smoked.

Treatment
➤ *Brief intervention and smoking cessation advice.* At its simplest, brief advice is defined as 'simply verbal instructions to stop smoking with or without added information about the harmful effects of smoking' (*ABC of Smoking Cessation*). Cost effective and achieves cessation in 1 out of 40 smokers.
➤ *Support Services.* Intensive behavioural support provided by smoking cessation counsellors. One in 13 smokers who are motivated and attend individual counselling are likely to quit.
➤ *Nicotine replacement therapy* (*NRT*): patches, gum, lozenges, inhalators, sub lingual tablets and nasal spray. Cochrane review suggests NRT leads to a doubling of cessation rates achieved by non-pharmacological intervention. Intensive support plus NRT produces 18% long-term abstinence.
➤ *Bupropion.* Atypical antidepressant. Inhibits reuptake of dopamine, noradrenaline and serotonin in the CNS and is a non-competitive nicotine receptor antagonist. Used with intensive behavioural support it is as effective as NRT. Should start 1 week before stopping smoking. Reduced dose recommended in older people. Contraindicated if history of seizures.
➤ *Varenicline*: nicotinic acetylcholine receptor partial agonist. Should be commenced 2 weeks prior to stopping smoking. Adverse effects commonly include nausea, headaches, insomnia and abnormal dreams. Reports of suicidal thoughts and behaviour exist.

PRESCRIPTION DRUGS
➤ Abuse of prescription drugs in older people covers a spectrum of problems, from single inappropriate use, use of drugs at higher doses and for longer periods than prescribed, use of prescribed drugs for another indication to recreational use and addiction.
➤ Most commonly involves benzodiazepines and opioid analgesics.
➤ Risk factors: female sex, social isolation, poor health status and multiple comorbidity, polypharmacy, previous substance use disorder, psychiatric illness.

Benzodiazepines
➤ Commonly prescribed for anxiety and sleep disorders.
➤ A study of benzodiazepine prescription to medical inpatients aged ≥65 in England and Wales suggested 65% of prescriptions were inappropriate.
➤ Long-term prescription of benzodiazepines (for as little as 2 months) may lead to physical dependence at therapeutic levels.
➤ Cause long-term effects on cognition, mood and behaviour.
➤ Withdrawal symptoms include recurrence of pre-treatment anxiety, rebound anxiety and insomnia, and a true withdrawal syndrome of irritability, agitation,

restlessness, insomnia, influenza-like symptoms, sensitivity to sound, touch or light, blurred vision, nightmares, hyper-reflexia, ataxia and rarely delirium, seizures, paranoid delusions, hallucinations or psychosis.

Opioid analgesics

➤ Commonly prescribed for pain relief, however, they can produce a feeling of euphoria when used non-medically.
➤ Opioid analgesics can cause physical and psychological dependence, sedation, impaired motor coordination, impaired cognitive and physical function.
➤ Withdrawal symptoms include restlessness, nausea and vomiting, dysphoria, aching muscles, diarrhoea, insomnia.

ILLICIT DRUGS

➤ Illicit drug use is rare in older people.
➤ The prevalence of lifetime experience of illicit drug use for people aged 65–9 is 24 per 1 000 people and for people aged 70–4 is 34 per 1 000. Cannabis and tranquillizers are the most common illicit drugs experienced.

FURTHER READING
Alcohol

Dar K. Alcohol use disorders in elderly people: fact or fiction. *Adv Psychiatr Treat.* 2006; **12**: 173–81.

Office for National Statistics. *General Household Survey 2007*. London: Office for National Statistics; 2009.

Patton A, Touquet R. *ABC of Alcohol*. Oxford: Blackwell; 2005.

University of Michigan Alcohol Research Center, *Michigan Alcohol Screening Test* (MAST-G). © The Regents of the University of Michigan, 1991.

Substance misuse

Britton J. *ABC of Smoking Cessation*. Oxford: Blackwell; 2004.

McGrath A, Crome P, Crome IB. Substance misuse in the older person. *Postgrad Med J.* 2005; **81**: 228–31.

Simoni-Wastila L, Yang HK. Psychoactive drug abuse in older adults. *Am J Geriatr Pharmacother.* 2006; **4**: 380–94.

Stead LF, Perera R, Bullen C, Mant D, Lancaster T. Nicotine replacement therapy for smoking cessation. *Cochrane Database of Systematic Reviews* 2008, Issue 1. Art. No.: CD000146. DOI: 10.1002/14651858.CD000146.pub3. http://www2.cochrane.org/reviews/en/ab000146.html

CHAPTER 19

Pressure ulcers

DEFINITION
➤ A pressure ulcer is an area of localised damage to skin and/or underlying tissue caused by pressure, shear, friction and/or a combination of these.[1]

STATISTICS
➤ Ill older people are at high risk.
➤ Inpatient prevalence ranges from 5–10%.
➤ Over 70% occur in those aged over 70.
➤ Increase mortality rate five-fold.
➤ Prolong hospital length of stay.
➤ Expensive to treat.
➤ A potential cause of litigation.
➤ Most can be prevented.

COMMON SITES
➤ Back of head.
➤ Ears.
➤ Shoulders.
➤ Rib cage.
➤ Elbows.
➤ Buttocks (sacrum/ischium).
➤ Legs (trochanters/malleoli).
➤ Heels.
➤ Toes.
➤ The areas affected depend on patient's position.

NATIONAL AND EUROPEAN PRESSURE ULCER ADVISORY PANEL CLASSIFICATION SYSTEM (2009)[2]
➤ Pressure ulcers are graded according to degree of tissue damage.
➤ Grade 1:
— non-blanchable erythema of intact skin
— discolouration, warmth, oedema or induration used as indicators, especially in darker skin.
➤ Grade 2:
— partial thickness skin loss involving epidermis and/or dermis
— presents clinically as an abrasion or blister.
➤ Grade 3:
— full-thickness skin loss involving damage to or necrosis of subcutaneous tissue

— may extend down to but not through fascia, bone, tendon or joint capsule.
➤ Grade 4:
    — extensive destruction, tissue necrosis or damage to muscle, bone or supporting structures with or without full-thickness skin loss.

RISK FACTORS
Intrinsic factors
➤ Reduced mobility, e.g. stroke/Parkinson's disease/arthritis.
➤ Impaired level of consciousness, e.g. neurological event/sedative medication.
➤ Acute illness, e.g. infection.
➤ Malnutrition.
➤ Dehydration.
➤ Sensory impairment, e.g. diabetes mellitus.
➤ Peripheral vascular disease.
➤ Moist skin, e.g. sweat/urine/faeces.
➤ Past history of pressure ulcers.

Extrinsic factors
➤ *Pressure.* Capillary occlusion compromises blood supply leading to tissue anoxia.
➤ *Shearing.* Superficial and deep tissue layers are forced in opposing directions, e.g. patient sliding down or being dragged up a bed or chair.
➤ *Friction.* Occurs when two surfaces move across each other, e.g. removal of superficial layers of skin through poor handling technique.

PREVENTION
➤ Patients should undergo a risk assessment by a trained member of staff within 6 hours of hospital admission.
➤ Pressure should be relieved with an appropriate support system.
➤ Skin should be inspected on a regular basis, paying particular attention to vulnerable areas.
➤ Frequency of repositioning should be determined by skin inspection.
➤ Staff should be trained in lifting techniques and the correct use of manual handling devices so that shear and friction damage can be avoided.
➤ Suitably trained staff, usually from the physiotherapy or occupational therapy departments, should advise regarding appropriate seating positions and aids.
➤ Adequate hydration and nutritional status should be maintained.
➤ Skin should be kept clean and dry.

TREATMENT
➤ Careful assessment of pressure ulcer with clear documentation of findings including cause, site, size, grade, depth, odour, presence of exudate/infection and sinus/fistula formation.
➤ Photograph wound if possible.
➤ Complete pressure relief with an appropriate device.
➤ Wound care (cleaning/prevention of infection/enhancement of granulation/ suitable dressings such as hydrocolloids) with close liaison with tissue viability specialist nurse.
➤ Consider antimicrobial therapy.
➤ Surgical referral for debridement may be necessary.
➤ Ensure adequate pain control.
➤ Optimise nutritional status (consider vitamin C and zinc).
➤ Minimise existing risk factors.

➤ All pressure ulcers graded 2 and above should be recorded locally as clinical incidents.

PRESSURE-RELIEVING DEVICES

➤ High-risk patients should be nursed on alternating pressure support mattresses: air-filled sacs inflate and deflate at different sites.
➤ Vulnerable but lower-risk patients can be placed on static support systems (high specification foam mattresses) that distribute body weight over a large area.
➤ Devices that should not be used include water-filled gloves, synthetic sheepskin and doughnut-type aids.

REFERENCES

1 European Pressure Ulcer Advisory Panel; 2003. www.epuap.org
2 European Pressure Ulcer Advisory Panel and National Pressure Ulcer Advisory Panel. *Clinical Guidelines on Prevention and Treatment of Pressure Ulcers*; 2009. www.epuap.org and www.npuap.org

FURTHER READING

National Institute for Health and Clinical Excellence. *Pressure Relieving Devices: the use of pressure-relieving devices for the prevention of pressure ulcers in primary and secondary care. NICE clinical guideline 7*. London: NIHCE; 2003. www.nice.org.uk/cg7
National Institute for Health and Clinical Excellence. *Pressure Ulcer Management: the prevention and treatment of pressure ulcers. NICE clinical guideline 29*. London: NIHCE; 2005. www.nice.org.uk/cg29

CHAPTER 20

Leg ulcers

- ➤ Approximately 120 000 people in the UK have leg ulcers.
- ➤ Commonly occur in older population.
- ➤ Functional capacity and quality of life can be adversely affected.
- ➤ Tissue Viability Services provide advice on the management of inpatients, including use of appropriate dressings, and follow patients up in an outpatient setting.
- ➤ There are three main types.

VENOUS ULCERS
- ➤ Account for 70–80% of leg ulcers.
- ➤ Occur as a result of chronic venous insufficiency.
- ➤ Usually present on the medial surface of the lower leg.
- ➤ Surrounding skin is often pigmented.
- ➤ Bacteria often colonise ulcers – antibiotic treatment should only be employed if evidence of active infection.
- ➤ External pressure assists healing by improving venous return and reducing swelling.
- ➤ Provided there is no arterial compromise, four-layer compression bandages should be applied.
- ➤ Once healed, patients should be encouraged to wear compression stockings (assistance may be required for frail community-dwelling older people).
- ➤ Venous ulcers can coexist with arterial ulcers (mixed).

ARTERIAL ULCERS
- ➤ 10% of leg ulcers are due to arterial insufficiency.
- ➤ The foot and lateral aspect of the lower leg are most commonly affected.
- ➤ The leg appears pale, dusky and cold with reduced/impalpable pulses.
- ➤ Intermittent claudication is a common presenting feature, although it may not be apparent in some older patients as comorbidity may restrict exercise tolerance.
- ➤ Rest pain may be a feature.
- ➤ Complications include cellulitis and osteomyelitis.
- ➤ Predisposing factors are smoking, hypertension, hypercholesterolaemia and diabetes mellitus.
- ➤ Risk factor modification plays an important role in prevention/treatment.
- ➤ Ankle:brachial pressure indices <0.7 indicate an arterial component.
- ➤ Suitable patients should be referred to a vascular surgeon.

DIABETIC ULCERS
- ➤ Approximately 5% of ulcers are related to diabetes mellitus.

➤ Often occur on the foot.
➤ Underlying atherosclerosis and consequent vascular insufficiency are common findings.
➤ Cellulitis should be treated aggressively with careful observation for signs of deep-seated infection.
➤ Poor control of glycaemia/blood pressure/lipids, continued smoking, inadequate foot care, sensory neuropathy and badly fitting shoes are contributing factors.
➤ Chiropody appointments every 3 months are advised.

FURTHER READING

Scottish Intercollegiate Guidelines Network. *The Care of Patients with Chronic Leg Ulcer. A National Clinical Guideline.* Edinburgh: SIGN; 1998. www.sign.ac.uk

CHAPTER 21

Clostridium difficile and methicillin-resistant Staphylococcus aureus (MRSA)

Rhodri Edwards

CLOSTRIDIUM DIFFICILE
Definition
➤ *Clostridium difficile* (*C. difficile*) is an anaerobic, gram-positive, spore-forming, toxin-producing bacillus.

Epidemiology and statistics
➤ Found in faecal flora of 3–5% of healthy adults.
➤ Found in stools of 10% of hospitalised adults without diarrhoea who receive antibiotics.
➤ Infects approximately 20% of hospitalised patients taking antibiotics.
➤ Predominately a problem of older people. Increasing age increases risk of infection and severity.
➤ In April–June 2009 the Health Protection Agency (HPA) reported 6 855 cases of *C. difficile*, 5 484 (80%) occurred in patients aged 65 or above.
➤ Reported cases of *C. difficile* in the UK are now falling. The HPA have reported a steady decline from 16 864 cases in April–June 2007 to 6 855 cases April–June 2009.

Pathogenesis
➤ Almost any antibiotic can cause *C. difficile* but those most commonly implicated are ampicillin, cephalosporins, fluoroquinolones and clindomycin.
➤ Transmission by faeco-oral route.
➤ *C. difficile* spores colonise large bowel, release two exotoxins (toxins A and B) which cause colitis and diarrhoea.
➤ *C. difficile* spores resist desiccation and can persist on hard surfaces for 5 months.
➤ Highly virulent BI/NAP1/027 strain commonly associated with outbreaks or epidemics such as at Stoke Mandeville Hospital.
➤ High titres of IgG against toxin A appear to be protective and a poor immunological response is associated with recurrent disease.

Risk factors
➤ Antibiotic use.
➤ Older age.
➤ Hospitalisation/institutional care (nursing homes/rehabilitation facilities).
➤ Caucasian race.
➤ Inflammatory bowel disease.
➤ Bowel surgery.
➤ Cancer chemotherapy.
➤ Presence of nasogastric tube.
➤ PPI therapy.

Clinical features
➤ Asymptomatic carrier.
➤ Diarrhoea.
➤ Fever.
➤ Abdominal discomfort or pain.
➤ Dehydration.
➤ Nausea and vomiting.
➤ Peritonitis.
➤ Sepsis syndrome.

Differential diagnosis
➤ Antibiotic-associated diarrhoea.
➤ Other infectious diarrhoea.
➤ Post-infectious irritable bowel syndrome.
➤ Coeliac disease.
➤ Inflammatory bowel disease.

Investigation
➤ Stool sample for faecal toxins – sensitive and specific.
➤ FBC (to detect leucocytosis with neutrophilia), U+E (to detect renal impairment), and LFTs (to detect hypoalbuminaemia).
➤ Abdominal radiograph – to exclude toxic megacolon.
➤ Sigmoidoscopy/colonoscopy if another cause of colitis suspected – not routinely recommended as risk of perforation.
➤ CT abdomen – in acute fulminant infection may help guide surgical management.

Markers of severity
➤ Severe diarrhoea – may be bloody and >12 stools/day.
➤ Pseudomembraneous colitis – only 50% have pseudomembranes.
➤ Ileus.
➤ Fever.
➤ Acute renal failure.
➤ Lactic acidosis.
➤ Hypoalbuminaemia.
➤ Peritonitis.

Management
Infection control and prevention
➤ Hand hygiene – hand washing with liquid soap or antimicrobial preparation and water since *C. difficile* spores can survive hand cleansing with alcohol-based gels.
➤ Isolation – physical isolation of patients in a single room with implementation of

barrier precautions including use of disposable gloves, gowns or aprons.
➤ Antibiotic stewardship – emphasising appropriate use of antibiotics particularly broad-spectrum agents.
➤ Environmental decontamination of rooms and equipment with sporicidal agents such as sodium hypochlorite.

Treatment
➤ Discontinue predisposing antibiotics wherever possible and observe clinical improvement.
➤ Hydration.
➤ Antibiotic treatment to ameliorate symptoms while allowing gradual restoration of normal gut flora:
  — metronidazole (400 mg orally tds for 10–14 days) – usual first line therapy. Can be given parenterally if required
  — vancomycin (125 mg orally qds for 10–14 days) – usually second line therapy although some advocate its use first line in severe infection. Note: parenteral vancomycin is not excreted into the colonic lumen and is not effective in treatment of *C. difficile*.
➤ Surgical referral for consideration of subtotal colectomy for fulminant disease – postoperative mortality 35–80%.
➤ Intravenous immunoglobulin.
➤ Probiotics – a meta-analysis supports prophylactic probiotics to reduce incidence of acute *C. difficile*. A recent Cochrane review (Loeb *et al.*) showed modest benefit of *Saccharomyces boulardii* as an adjuvant to antibiotics.

Recurrent disease
➤ After successful initial treatment, 15–30% of patients have a symptomatic recurrence after stopping antibiotics.
➤ May be re-infection or incomplete eradication.
➤ Relapse rate is higher in older patients and patients with a previous history of *C. difficile*.
➤ First recurrence can be treated with a further course of metronidazole.
➤ Further relapses may require prolonged pulsed and reducing courses of vancomycin.
➤ Other therapeutic options include intravenous immunoglobulin, binding resins such as cholestyramine, rifampicin and faecal enemas (unpopular for reasons of diginity and practicality).

METHICILLIN-RESISTANT *STAPHYLOCOCCUS AUREUS*
Definition
MRSA refers to isolates of *Staphylococcus aureus* (*S. aureus*), a gram-positive cocci, resistant to β-lactam antibiotics including penicillins and cephalosporins.

Epidemiology and statistics
➤ 10–20% of general population are persistent carriers of *S. aureus* and 30–50% are intermittent carriers.
➤ 3% of the population are colonised with MRSA.
➤ MRSA is predominately a problem of older people.
➤ Approximately 25% of hospital staff are carriers of *S. aureus*. A review of multiple studies suggested the prevalence of MRSA amongst health workers is 4.6% – a higher prevalence noted in healthcare workers caring for geriatric patients 5.3%, doctors 8.0% and nursing staff 7.4%.

➤ MRSA has a higher prevalence in institutional care facilities with reported rate varying from 4.7% and 17%.
➤ Significant geographical variation: the Netherlands <1%, Germany 19%, France 33%, the UK 40% and USA 50%.
➤ MRSA is endemic in many UK hospitals.
➤ Most recently, a decline in MRSA infection has been noted in several European countries. In the UK, reported cases of MRSA bacteraemia fell by 34.1% between the financial year 2007/8 and 2008/9 (Health Protection Agency).
➤ Community acquired MRSA is increasingly recognised as a significant problem.
➤ MRSA represents a significant burden on UK health resources – estimated at £1 billion per year.

Microbiology
➤ Resistance to methicillin is mediated by an altered membrane-bound enzyme; penicillin-binding protein 2a encoded by the *mec*A gene.
➤ Many strains of MRSA are resistant to multiple other classes of antimicrobial agents including macrolides and quinolones.
➤ Emerging strains have reduced susceptibility to glycopeptides, i.e. vancomycin intermediate *S. aurues* (VISA)/gycopeptide intermediate *S. aureus* (GISA) and vancomycin resistant *S. aureus* (VRSA). VRSA has not been isolated in the UK and numbers remain low.

MRSA colonisation
➤ Colonisation is instrumental in the pathogenesis of MRSA.
➤ Most patients are colonised prior to infection.
➤ Primary reservoir of *S. aureus* is anterior nares but can be isolated from multiple sites (throat, groin, perineum).
➤ 80% of cases of *S. aureus* bacteraemia are due to the strain isolated from the patient's anterior nares.
➤ Majority of carriers are asymptomatic. Approximately one third will develop a MRSA infection.

Risk factors for MRSA colonisation
➤ Previous colonisation or infection with MRSA.
➤ Frequent readmissions to hospital.
➤ Direct inter-hospital transfers.
➤ Recent in patient at a hospital abroad or hospitals in the UK with high rates of MRSA.
➤ Living in residential care facilities.
➤ Prior antibiotic use.
➤ Intravenous drug users (IVDU), patients with HIV, patients with skin or soft tissue infection and members of professional contact sports teams.
➤ *S. aureus* colonisation is more prevalent in patients with type I diabetes, dermatological conditions such as eczema, patients undergoing haemodialysis and patients with HIV.

Mode of transmission
➤ Infected or colonised patient acts as a reservoir; less commonly healthcare workers.
➤ Patient-to-patient transmission primarily occurs via exposure to the hands of healthcare workers.

➤ *S. aureus* can survive for months in dry, relatively hostile environments, e.g. door handles.
➤ Other routes of transmission include contamination from the environment (floors, medical equipment, hospital furniture, patient charts, tourniquets) and airborne contamination (particularly relevant to patients with tracheostomies and those in burns units).

Clinical syndromes
➤ MRSA is associated with range of infections – signs and symptoms vary with site of infection.

Risk factors for MRSA infection
➤ Previous colonisation or infection with MRSA.
➤ Prolonged and recurrent hospital admissions.
➤ Inter-hospital transfers.
➤ Living in institutional care facilities.
➤ Prior and repeated antibiotic exposure.
➤ Chronic illness, debilitation and multiple comorbidities.
➤ Indwelling devices (intravascular device, urinary catheter, ET [endotracheal tube], tracheotomy).
➤ ITU admission.
➤ Ventilation.
➤ Enteral feeding.
➤ Skin ulcers and dermatological conditions such as eczema.
➤ Surgery.
➤ IVDU.
➤ Presence of immunosuppressive conditions.
➤ Units such as ITU, transplantation centres, cardiothoracic, orthopaedic, trauma, vascular surgery and renal units are at high risk of serious MRSA infections.

Bacteraemia
➤ Associated with increased mortality – compared with methicillin-sensitive *S. aureus*, MRSA bacteraemia has a relative risk of 2.12.
➤ Increased mortality is associated with increasing age, non-removable foci of infection and underlying cardiac, neurological and respiratory disease.
➤ The most common sources of MRSA bacteraemia are intravenous catheters and intravascular devices, skin and soft tissue infections and ventilator-associated pneumonia.
➤ One third of patients with MRSA bacteraemia have evidence of metastatic infection (involving the heart valves, intervertebral discs, intra-abdominal organs, bones and joints).
➤ To diagnose bacteraemia and identify source of infection it is recommended:
    — serial blood culture every 48–72 hours
    — radiological imaging and echocardiography (including transoesophageal echocardiography).
➤ Management should focus on establishing the source of infection, initiating appropriate antibiotic therapy and a high index of suspicion for metastatic infection.

Endocarditis
➤ *S. aureus* endocarditis accounts for 25–35% of endocarditis – in one study, 55% of patients with *S. aureus* bacteraemia had evidence of endocarditis at post mortem

in the absence of clinical suspicion. Another study showed 25% of patients had evidence of endocarditis on transoesophageal echocardiogram without clinical or transthoracic echocardiogram findings.
➤ Risk groups: IVDU, older people, patients with prosthetic valves and hospitalised patients.
➤ IVDU associated with right-sided vegetations.
➤ Left-sided MRSA endocarditis is more common in older patients and patients with chronic conditions. It is associated with high incidence of embolic and neurological complications and a high mortality rate (20–44%).

Community-associated MRSA
➤ Community-associated MRSA (CA-MRSA) caused by a different strain to hospital-acquired infection has been increasingly reported since the mid-1990s. It is more common in the USA.
➤ It is mainly been described in context of skin and soft tissue infections, however, reports of sepsis and necrotising pneumonia exist.
➤ CA-MRSA is resistant to fewer antibiotics, produces different toxins and has different genetic constitution mediating resistance to methicillin.

Management
Infection control and prevention
➤ *Surveillance* as part of an infection control programme involves collecting, analysing, interpreting and disseminating data available on MRSA colonisation and infection to guide public health practice and infection control.
  — *Antibiotic stewardship* – avoidance of inappropriate or excessive antibiotic therapy, ensuring antibiotics are given at correct dosage and for appropriate duration, appropriate use of glycopeptides antibiotics, clinically appropriate use of broad-spectrum antibiotics (third generation cephalosporins and fluoroquinolones).
➤ *Screening* for MRSA carriage to help guide interventions such as isolation, cohorting and decolonisation.

Prevention and control measures
➤ Hand hygiene – thorough washing and/or a 70% alcohol hand rub preparation.
➤ Isolation/cohorting – physical isolation of patients either in a single room or as a cohort. Disposable gloves, aprons or gowns should be worn.
➤ Environmental decontamination. Enhanced cleaning of facilities (including curtains and linen) and decontamination of equipment is important. Cleaning of surfaces frequently touched, e.g. monitors, keyboards, is an important consideration.
➤ Patient movement minimised to reduce risk of cross infection.

Elimination of carriage
➤ Decolonisation generally involves topical agents such as nasal ointment and body wash/shampoo to eradicate/reduce nasal and skin carriage.
➤ Natural history of MRSA carriage without treatment: ~40% remain persistent carriers particularly if skin breaks are present.
➤ The British Society of Antimicrobial Chemotherapy Guidelines (2008) recommend mupirocin with a systemically active agent for treatment and clearance of mupirocin-susceptible MRSA in patients with carriage or possible infection of soft tissue lesions. This recommendation aimed to improve clearance rates beyond those with nasal or topical mupirocin alone.

Agents used

➤ Mupirocin – a topical anti-staphylococcal agent that inhibits RNA and protein synthesis:
  — nasal topical application of mupirocin for 4–7 days is most effective treatment for eradicating MRSA
  — established and increasing resistance to mupirocin is a problem
  — repeated and prolonged used of mupirocin is not recommended.
➤ Various combinations of rifampicin, tetracyclines, mupirocin and both topical and oral fusidic acid.
➤ Skin decolonisation using 4% chlorhexidine body wash/shampoo, 7.5% povidone-iodine or 2% triclosan is useful in eradicating or suppressing skin colonisation for short periods, such as preoperatively.

Treatment of MRSA infections[1]

Chloramphenicol	CNS infections
Clindamycin	Skin and soft tissue infections, bone and joint infections
Co-trimoxazole	Skin and soft tissue infections
Daptomycin	Bacteraemia, skin and soft tissue infections
Fusidic acid	Skin and soft tissue infections, adjunct for bone infections
Linzolid	Pneumonia, serious soft tissue infection, bactraemia, resistant infections (GISA,VRSA)
Quinupristin/dalfopristin	Reserve drug for GISA and GRSA infections
Rifampicin	Bone and joint infection, skin and soft tissue infections, eradication therapy, adjunct treatment in management of prosthetic infections
Teicoplanin	Serious soft tissue infection, bacteraemia
Tetracyclines	Skin and soft tissue infections, UTI, eradication of carriage
Trimethoprim	UTI, other use in combination
Vancomycin	Bacteraemia, soft tissue infection, bone infection

Adapted from Guidelines (2008) for the prophylaxis and treatment of methicillin-resistant *Staphylococcus aureus* (MRSA) infections in the United Kingdom. *J Antimicrob Chemo*. 2009; **63**: 849–61.

REFERENCE

1 Gould FK, Brindle R, Chadwick PR, Fraise AP, Hill S, Nathwani D, Ridgway GL, Spry MJ, Warren RE. Guidelines (2008) for the prophylaxis and treatment of methicillin-resistant *Staphylococcus aureus* (MRSA) infections in the United Kingdom. *J Antimicrob Chemo*. 2009; **63**: 849–61.

FURTHER READING

Leffler DA, Lamont JT. Treatment of *Clostridium difficile*-associated disease. *Gastroenterology*. 2009; **136**: 1899–1912

Loeb M, Malin C, Walker-Dilks C, Eady A. Antimicrobial drugs for treating methicillin-resistant *Staphlococcus aureus* colonization. (Cochrane Review). In: The Cochrane Library, Issue 3. Chichester: John Wiley & Son; 2003.

Lowy FD. *Staphylococcus aureus* infections. *N Eng J Med*. 1998; **339**: 520–32.

McFee RB, Abdelsayed GG. Clostridium difficile. *Dis Mon*. 2009; **55**: 439–70.

Health Protection Agency. *Quarterly Analyses: mandatory MRSA bacteraemia and* Clostridium difficile *infections (July 2007 to September 2009)*. London: Health Protection Agency; 3 December 2009. www.hpa.org.uk/web/HPAwebFile/HPAweb_C/1259152023516

Health Protection Agency. *Quarterly Epidemiological Commentary: mandatory MRSA bacteraemia and* Clostridium difficile *infection (October 2007 to December 2009)*. London: Health Protection Agency; 19 March 2010. www.hpa.org.uk/web/HPAwebFile/HPAweb_C/1267551242367

CHAPTER 22

HIV in older people

Rhodri Edwards

STATISTICS

➤ Older patients in the context of HIV infection have been considered as people over 50 years of age.

➤ The Health Protection Agency (HPA) estimated 77 400 people were living with HIV in the UK at the end of 2007 of whom 28% were unaware of their infection.

➤ The number of people over the age of 50 accessing HIV care increased from 1 679 in 1998 to 8 722 in 2007. In 2007 older adults represented 15% of all people accessing HIV care. (Health Protection Agency).

➤ In 2008 the HPA reported 7 298 new HIV diagnoses. 11% were in people over 50. (Health Protection Agency – unadjusted statistics).

➤ In 2008 the HPA reported 3 717 (1 435 male, 2 282 female) new HIV infections as a result of heterosexual contact. 11.7% were in people over 50. (Health Protection Agency – unadjusted statistics). Previous analysis suggests three quarters of these infections were acquired abroad mainly affecting the black African population who acquired their infection in sub-Saharan Africa. However, the number of persons infected by heterosexual contact within the UK is rising significantly.

➤ 33% of new diagnoses of HIV in 2008 were among men who have sex with men. 10.5% of these were aged over 50. New HIV diagnoses among gay men continue to rise, increasing from 1 575 in 2000 to 2 433 in 2008 and most of these infections were probably acquired in the UK. HIV surveillance data from 2000–07 suggests 44% of newly diagnosed older gay men were infected with HIV when ≥ 50. (Health Protection Agency – unadjusted statistics).

➤ Very few older people newly acquire HIV from intravenous drug use in the UK.

➤ Gay men and black African heterosexual men and women account for 80% of people living with HIV in the UK.

➤ Due to highly active antiretroviral treatment (HAART) people are living longer with HIV infection. By 2015, ~50% of people living with HIV will be over 50.

POPULATIONS OF OLDER PEOPLE LIVING WITH HIV

➤ *The ageing cohort* – people diagnosed with HIV under age of 50 who are living longer due to HAART.

➤ *Late diagnosis* – people diagnosed with HIV over the age of 50. People may have been infected with HIV in their 30s or 40s but diagnosed later. Late diagnosis with lower CD4 counts is more common in older people.

➤ *Late seroconverters* – people infected over age of 50. Raises important questions about HIV risk behaviours in older people.

SPECIFIC CONSIDERATIONS FOR HIV RISK IN OLDER PEOPLE

➤ Older people are sexually active and some are intravenous drugs users putting them at risk of HIV transmission.

➤ Changes in society such as increased divorce rates combined with increased longevity increase the opportunity for older people to acquire new sexual partners.

➤ Greater travel and tourism provides increased opportunity for causal and/or commercial sex in high risk areas.

➤ Postmenopausal women who do not need barrier contraception for birth control often neglect the risk of sexually transmitted infection.

➤ Vaginal dryness in older women may increase risk of infection.

➤ The Internet provides a novel way for older people to meet new partners. However, older gay men are less likely to serosort (the practice of identifying social and sexual partners based on HIV status) on the Internet than younger men.

➤ Pharmacological advances with Viagra mean more older people can have sex more frequently and for longer.

➤ Screening strategies have traditionally targeted IVDU, gay men, pregnant women and people attending genitourinary medicine clinics. HIV testing needs to target the older population as they are more likely to remain undiagnosed at present.

➤ Older people with HIV have a higher prevalence of drug and alcohol use.

➤ Older people often have developed primary caring responsibilities for others affected with HIV (often their children and grandchildren), particularly in the developing world.

HIV DISEASE AND CD4 COUNT

CD4 <350 cells/mm3	CD4 <200 cells/mm3	CD4 <100 cells/mm3
Pulmonary tuberculosis	Pneumocystis jirovecii pneumonia	Cerebral toxoplasmosis
Pneumococcal pneumonia	Oesophageal candidiasis	HIV-associated dementia
Herpes zoster	Mucocutaneous herpes simplex	Cryptococcal meningitis
Oropharyngeal candidiasis	Miliary or extrapulmonary tuberculosis	Progressive multifocal leucoencephalopathy
Oral hairy leucoplakia	Cryptosporidium	Non-Hodgkin's lymphoma
Extra-intestinal salmonellosis	HIV-wasting	Cytomegalovirus retinitis or colitis
HIV associated idiopathic thrombocytopenic purpura	Microsporidium	Disseminated Mycobacterium avium intracellulare
Cervical intra epithelial neoplasia II–III	Peripheral neuropathy	Primary central nervous system lymphoma
Lymphoid interstitial pneumonitis		
Karposi's sarcoma		

AIDS DEFINING ILLNESSES

Oesophageal candidiasis	Progressive multifocal leucoencephalopathy
Cryptococcal meningitis	Recurrent non-typhi *Salmonella* septicaemia
Chronic cryptosporidium diarrhoea	Cerebral toxoplasmosis
Cytomegalovirus retinitis or colitis	Karposi's sarcoma
Chronic mucocutaneous herpes simplex	Non-Hodgkin's lymphoma
Disseminated Mycobacterium avium intracellulare	Primary cerebral lymphoma
Coccidioidomycosis: disseminated or extrapulmonary	Invasive cervical carcinoma
Histoplasmosis: disseminated or extrapulmonary	HIV-associated wasting
Miliary or extrapulmonary tuberculosis	HIV-associated dementia
Pneumocystis jirovecii pneumonia	

HAART TREATMENT

UK Guidelines recommend use of two nucleoside analogues (Zidovudine [AZT], Didanosine [ddI], Stavudine [d4t], Lamivudine [3TC], Abacavir [ABC], Emtricitabine) plus with a boosted protease inhibitor (Saquinavir, Indinavir, Nelfinavir, Amprenavir, Ritonavir, Atazanavir, Darunavir, Fosamprenavir, Tipranavir) or a non-nucleoside reverse transcriptase inhibitor (Nevirapine, Efavirenz, Etravirine).

However, it is important to note that:

➤ older people may be more likely to develop drug toxicity
➤ older people more likely to have comorbidities complicating use of HAART
➤ most randomised controlled trials of antiretroviral drugs excluded older patients and those with comorbidities
➤ deciding to commence HAART needs a careful evaluation of preserving immunological function and the higher risks of complication and toxicity from treatment in older people
➤ management should always be led by an HIV physician.

FURTHER READING

Auerbach JD. HIV/AIDS and aging: intervention for older adults. *JAIDS*. 2003; **33**: S57–8.

Elford J, Ibrahim F, Bukutu C, Anderson J. Over fifty and living with HIV in London. *Sex Transm Infect*. 2008; **84**: 468–72.

Health Protection Agency. *HIV in the United Kingdom: 2008 report*. London: Health Protection Agency; November 2008. www.hpa.org.uk/web/HPAwebFile/HPAweb_C/1227515298354

Health Protection Agency. *Testing Times: HIV and Other Sexually Transmitted Infections in the United Kingdom: 2007*. London: Health Protection Agency; 23 November 2007. www.hpa.org.uk/web/HPAwebFile/HPAweb_C/1203496897276

Health Protection Agency. *Quarterly Epidemiological Commentary: mandatory MRSA bacteraemia and* Clostridium difficile *infection (October 2007 to December 2009)*. London: Health Protection Agency; 2010. www.hpa.org.uk/web/HPAwebFile/HPAweb_C/1267551242367

CHAPTER 23

Hypothermia

DEFINITION
➤ Core body temperature <35°C.

CLASSIFICATION
➤ Mild   35–32.2°C.
➤ Moderate   32.2–28°C.
➤ Severe   <28°C.

STATISTICS
➤ Mortality rates for older people increase during winter months.
➤ Approximately 40 000 excess winter deaths occur in England and Wales each year.
➤ Majority of these are attributed to vascular (myocardial infarction/stroke) and respiratory causes.
➤ Cold weather induces haemoconcentration, which predisposes to thrombogenesis and impairs the body's responses to infection.
➤ Hypothermia is the certified cause of death in only around 300 cases per annum (and so more likely to be a secondary event).

RISK FACTORS FOR HYPOTHERMIA
➤ Medical illness (e.g. fall with long lie).
➤ Alcohol.
➤ Sedative medication.
➤ Poor heating.
➤ Inadequate finances.

PRESENTATION
Mild
➤ Lethargy.
➤ Irritability.
➤ Confusion.
➤ Loss of fine motor coordination.
➤ Impaired judgement.
➤ Shivering.
➤ Tachycardia.
➤ Tachypnoea.

Moderate
➤ Reduced conscious level.

➤ Bradycardia.
➤ Arrhythmias (atrial fibrillation/ventricular tachycardia-fibrillation).
➤ Reduced respiratory rate.
➤ Oliguria.

Severe

➤ Coma.
➤ Arrhythmias (ventricular fibrillation/asystole).

MANAGEMENT

➤ Airway/breathing/circulation.
➤ Treat any precipitating underlying causes.
➤ Rewarming methods can include:
  — removal of wet clothing
  — blankets
  — hot air blankets
  — warm humidified oxygen
  — warm intravenous fluids.
➤ Prevention:
  — risk factor modification
  — education
  — care alarm
  — adequate home heating
  — financial advice and support
  — winter visits for high risk individuals.

CHAPTER 24

Hearing impairment/tinnitus

HEARING IMPAIRMENT
Definition
➤ Hearing loss is the total or partial inability to hear sound in one or both ears.
➤ Presbycusis (age-related hearing loss) is the progressive loss of the ability to hear high frequencies, e.g. speech.

Statistics
➤ Nine million people in the UK have some degree of hearing impairment.
➤ Hearing loss is the most common sensory impairment in older people.
➤ In 2001 in UK:
— 50 000 people were registered deaf
— 144 000 were registered hard of hearing (62% aged over 75).
➤ Prevalence increases with age: 25% of population by 65 years, 50% by 75 years and 75% by 80 years.

Investigation
➤ Weber's test: a test to determine the nature of unilateral hearing loss in which a vibrating tuning fork is held against the forehead at the midline. Conduction deafness is indicated if the sound is heard more loudly in the affected ear and nerve deafness is indicated if it is heard more loudly in the normal ear.
➤ Rinne's test: a test to determine the ability to hear a vibrating tuning fork when it is held next to the ear and when it is placed on the mastoid process. Diminished hearing activity through air and somewhat heightened hearing activity through bone are suggestive of conductive deafness.
➤ Whisper test: a basic first-line test of hearing where the clinician whispers a number in one of the patient's ears whilst occluding the other ear, and asks the patient to repeat the number.
➤ Auroscopy.
➤ Referral for audiometry.

Classification of hearing impairment
1 Conductive deafness
— impaired sound transmission through external canal and middle ear
— common causes include obstruction of external auditory meatus, e.g. wax/discharge/foreign bodies, perforation of eardrum and otosclerosis.
2 Sensorineural deafness
— secondary to cochlear or retro-cochlear pathology

— causes include presbycusis, Meniere's disease, drugs, e.g. gentamicin, and infection.

Management of presbycusis
➤ No known cure.
➤ Hearing aids may help.
➤ Lip reading and using visual cues may aid communication.

Hearing aids
➤ Electronic devices consisting of a microphone, amplifier, loud speaker and battery.
➤ 1.4 million people use prescribed hearing aids in England and Wales.

Communication tips
➤ Have the listener's attention.
➤ Ensure the face of the speaker is well-illuminated.
➤ Reduce background noise.
➤ Maintain an optimal distance of 1 metre.
➤ Use a low-pitched voice.
➤ Speak slowly and clearly rather than shouting.
➤ Reword a misunderstood phrase instead of repeating.

Consequences of poor hearing
➤ Social isolation.
➤ Depression.
➤ Hazard risk, e.g. fire, traffic.

TINNITUS
Definition
➤ A sensation of sound arising in the head or ears.
➤ Note that musical noise, words or meaningful sounds are not tinnitus and may be indicative of a psychiatric or neurological disorder.

Prevalence
➤ Increases with age – 14.5% are over 40 years of age and 22% are over 60 years of age.
➤ Majority of patients have some degree of deafness.

Aetiology
➤ In majority of cases cause is unknown.
➤ Meniere's disease.
➤ Acoustic trauma.
➤ Chronic otitis media.
➤ Drug induced – aminoglycosides, chloramphenicol.
➤ Otosclerosis.
➤ Post-middle ear surgery.
➤ Pulsatile tinnitus – due to haemodynamic disorders.
➤ Involuntary contractions of palatal muscles, tympani or stapedal muscles – the 'clicking noise' may also be heard by others.

Management

➤ Majority require assurance only after full assessment and investigations have been performed and a full explanation provided.

➤ Hearing aids for those with hearing loss may also mask tinnitus.

➤ Maskers.

➤ Electrical stimulation/suppression.

➤ Biofeedback.

➤ Support group – British Tinnitus Association.

➤ Antidepressants if depression present.

CHAPTER 25

Visual impairment

STATISTICS
➤ UK figures for 2008:
  — 156 300 people registered partially sighted
  — 153 000 people registered blind
  — 64% of blind and 66% of partially-sighted people are aged over 75 years
  — 30% of those aged over 65 years are estimated to be visually impaired in both eyes
  — 70% of such cases are potentially remediable
  — The incidence of visual impairment is expected to increase by 35% by 2020 as the older population grows.

EYE TESTS
➤ Free NHS eye examinations are available to the over-60s.
➤ The demand for NHS sight tests will rise by 20% over the next 20 years as the population aged over 60 increases.
➤ NHS provides a domiciliary service for those who are housebound or resident in long-term care facilities.
➤ Advisable every 2 years in older people and annually in people with diabetes mellitus.
➤ Active screening for visual loss should be part of the routine assessment process using a Snellen chart to test visual acuity as a minimum.

REGISTRATION OF SIGHT LOSS
➤ Many older people eligible for blind and partially-sighted status are not registered.
➤ Blind registration entitles people to financial and other benefits.
➤ The Royal National Institute of Blind People (RNIB)[1] can provide useful information to patients and their carers.

CONSEQUENCES OF POOR VISION
➤ Accidents (see driving standards).
➤ Falls.
➤ Fractures (especially hip).
➤ Reduced functional status and increased dependency.
➤ Poor quality of life.
➤ Social isolation.
➤ Depression.

COMMON CAUSES OF VISUAL IMPAIRMENT
Refractive errors
➤ More than 30% of visual impairment in older people is due solely to refractive errors.
➤ Can be simply corrected with glasses.

Cataracts
➤ 25% of the over-75s are affected.
➤ The most common treatable cause of impaired vision.
➤ Cataract extraction is the most common elective surgical procedure performed in older people with 105 000 NHS operations each year.

Glaucoma
➤ Prevalence in patients aged over 75 years is approximately 5%.
➤ Early detection important.
➤ Results in optic nerve damage with consequent sight loss and blindness.
➤ Chronic open angle glaucoma is the most common form.
➤ Intraocular pressure can be reduced with topical miotic agents or surgery in some cases.

Age-related macular degeneration
➤ The most important cause of irremediable visual loss in older people.
➤ Over 500 000 people are affected in the UK.
➤ Characterised by loss of central vision.
➤ Two forms: dry (non-exudative) and wet (exudative).
➤ Dry form results from cellular debris accumulation (drusen) between choroid and retina.
➤ Wet form occurs secondary to choroidal neovascularisation.
➤ Amsler Grid Test can be used in detection and monitoring.
➤ Management options include photocoagulation and anti-angiogenic therapy for the wet form and low vision aids for the dry type.

Diabetic retinopathy
➤ Consequences can be reduced through good glycaemic control and early detection.
➤ Laser treatment can be used in proliferative disease.

NATIONAL EYE CARE SERVICES STEERING GROUP (2004)[2]
➤ Evidence-based care pathways for the management of low vision, cataracts, glaucoma and age-related macular degeneration have been developed.
➤ Aims to promote a more efficient service.
➤ Supports integration of eye care services across primary and secondary care.
➤ Expands the role of optometrists, e.g. direct referrals to hospital eye service.

UK VISION STRATEGY[3]
➤ Aims:
— to improve the eye health of people of the UK
— to eliminate avoidable sight loss and deliver excellent support to those with visual impairment
— to enhance the inclusion, participation and independence of blind and partially sighted people.

VISUAL STANDARDS IN DRIVING (DRIVING AND VEHICLE LICENSING AUTHORITY)[4]

➤ Drivers must be able to read, in good light with the aid of corrective lenses, if necessary, a registration mark fixed to a motor vehicle containing letters and figures 79.4 mm high at a distance of 20.5 m (equivalent to binocular visual acuity of 6/10).

➤ An adequate field of vision is necessary.

REFERENCES

1 Royal National Institute of the Blind. www.rnib.org.uk
2 National Eye Care Services Steering Group. London: Department of Health; 2004. www.dh.gov.uk
3 UK Vision Strategy. www.vision2020uk.org.uk/ukvisionstrategy
4 Driver and Vehicle Licensing Agency. www.dft.gov.uk/dvla

FURTHER READING

National Institute for Health and Clinical Excellence. *Glaucoma: diagnosis and management of chronic open angle glaucoma and ocular hypertension. NICE clinical guideline 85.* London: NIHCE; 2009. www.nice.org.uk/cg85

CHAPTER 26

Hypertension

AGE, HYPERTENSION AND CARDIOVASCULAR RISK

➤ Of Europe's population 20% are aged over 65 years.
➤ The 'old old' population (over 80 years) is increasing most rapidly.
➤ Cardiovascular disease is the single most frequent cause of death in the over-65s, is responsible for considerable morbidity and has significant cost implications for the NHS and social services.
➤ The link between hypertension and increased cardiovascular risk in older people is well known.
➤ Hypertension continues to be a significant health problem in older people.
➤ In the United Kingdom more than 50% of the 10 million people over 65 years old are hypertensive.
➤ Older hypertensive patients are now seen as an important target group who appear to benefit from antihypertensive treatment in terms of improved outcomes.
➤ Intervention trials have demonstrated that antihypertensive treatment in older patients can reduce the incidence of stroke by 30%, coronary heart disease by 20% and all vascular deaths by nearly 25%.
➤ An aggressive approach to blood pressure lowering is warranted up to and beyond the age of 80, particularly in those at increased cardiovascular risk.
➤ The absolute benefit from treatment in older people is much larger than that for younger patients with hypertension because of their higher absolute risk.

ISOLATED SYSTOLIC HYPERTENSION (ISH)

➤ A distinct pathological entity arising from reduced vascular compliance resulting in systolic blood pressures (SBP) >160 mmHg and diastolic blood pressures (DBP) <90 mmHg.
➤ The rise in SBP causes left ventricular hypertrophy and the reduction in DBP may compromise coronary blood flow.
➤ Prevalence increases with age (8% in the over-60s and 25% in those aged over 80 years).
➤ The Framingham Heart Study showed that among hypertensive people aged over 65 years, 70% had ISH rather than combined systolic and diastolic hypertension.
➤ A better predictor of cardiovascular events than DBP.

BRITISH HYPERTENSION SOCIETY GUIDELINES (2004)[1]

➤ Routine investigations should include:
  — urinalysis
  — serum electrolytes and creatinine

— plasma glucose
— serum total:HDL cholesterol.

➤ 12-lead ECG.
➤ Lifestyle modification should be encouraged in all hypertensive and borderline hypertensive people:
— weight loss
— regular exercise
— reduced use of salt
— increased intake of fruit and vegetables
— reduced caffeine intake
— limited alcohol consumption
— reduced total/saturated fat intake.

➤ Initiate antihypertensive drug therapy in people with sustained SBP >160 mmHg or sustained DBP >100 mmHg.
➤ Decide on treatment in people with sustained SBP between 140 and 159 mmHg or sustained DBP between 90 and 99 mmHg according to the presence or absence of target organ damage, cardiovascular disease or a 10-year cardiovascular disease risk of more than 20%.
➤ In non-diabetic hypertensive people, optimal BP targets are SBP <140 mmHg and DBP <85 mmHg.
➤ In people with diabetes, start antihypertensive treatment if SBP is sustained above 140 mmHg or DBP is sustained over 90 mmHg.
➤ In hypertensive people with diabetes, chronic renal disease or established cardiovascular disease, optimal SBP and DBP readings are <130 mmHg and <80 mmHg respectively.
➤ Combination therapy will be required to achieve recommended BP targets in many cases.
➤ Other drugs that reduce cardiovascular risk should be considered:
— aspirin for secondary prevention of cardiovascular disease and primary prevention in treated hypertensive patients >50 years who have a 10-year risk of more than 20%
— statins for hypertensive people with established cardiovascular disease irrespective of total and LDL cholesterol levels. Statins should also be prescribed for primary prevention in people with high blood pressure and a 10-year cardiovascular disease risk of more than 20%.

ANTIHYPERTENSIVE DRUG THERAPY

➤ In 2006 the National Institute for Health and Clinical Excellence (NICE) and the British Hypertension Society (BHS) updated the 2004 BHS guideline with respect to drug therapy for hypertensive people over the age of 55:[2]
— Step: 1 C or D
           2 A & C or A & D
           3 A & C & D
           4 add further diuretic therapy or an α-blocker or a β-blocker/consider specialist referral

Key:
A ACE-inhibitors/angiotensin II receptor antagonists
C Calcium channel blockers
D Diuretics

HYVET STUDY: TREATMENT OF HYPERTENSION IN PATIENTS 80 YEARS OF AGE OR OLDER (2008)[3]

Provides evidence that treatment of hypertension in the very old (to achieve a target of 150/80 mmHg) with sustained release indapamide with or without perindopril, is associated with reduced risks of death from stroke, death from any cause and heart failure.

MANAGEMENT PROBLEMS IN THE OLDER HYPERTENSIVE PATIENT

➤ Older hypertensives represent a special group with particular needs and antihypertensive prescribing can be both a clinical and practical challenge.

➤ Older people show greater blood pressure variability so it is important to take multiple measurements on several occasions to confirm the diagnosis.

➤ Lying and standing recordings should be taken at the start of treatment and during the follow-up phase because of the high prevalence of postural hypotension in this age group.

➤ A regime for the older hypertensive patient should ideally be:
  — based on recommended guidelines
  — appropriate to comorbidities
  — suitable for once-daily dosing
  — well-tolerated
  — unlikely to prompt non-compliance
  — cost-effective.

➤ Most patients will have comorbidities dictating which agents should be used first line, e.g. ACE inhibitors or angiotensin II receptor antagonists in hypertensive patients with diabetes or those with cardiac failure or a history of stroke.

➤ More than one drug will often be required to achieve control.

➤ Coexisting diseases preclude certain drug choices.

➤ Polypharmacy can lead to drug interactions, drug-related side-effects and medication non-concordance.

➤ Salt restriction is difficult to practice in view of diminished taste sensation.

➤ Compliance with weight loss and diet restrictions is often unsuccessful.

➤ Disturbance in cognitive function may affect drug compliance.

REFERENCES

1 Williams B *et al.* Guidelines for the management of hypertension: report of the fourth working party of the British Hypertension Society, 2004 (BHS-IV). *J Hum Hypertens.* 2004; **18**: 139–85. Available at: www.bhsoc.org/pdfs/Summary%20Guidelines%202004.pdf (accessed 25 May 2010).

2 National Institute for Health and Clinical Excellence. *Hypertension: management in adults in primary care: pharmacological update: NICE clinical guideline 34.* London: NIHCE; 2006. Available at: www.nice.org.uk/cg34 (accessed 25 May 2010).

3 Beckett NS *et al.* Treatment of hypertension in patients 80 years of age or older. *N Engl J Med.* 2008; **358**: 1887–98. Available at: http://content.nejm.org/cgi/content/full/NEJMoa0801369 (accessed 25 May 2010).

CHAPTER 27

Heart failure

DEFINITION (NICE 2003)[1]

➤ Heart failure is a complex syndrome that can result from any structural or functional disorder that impairs the ability of the heart to function as a pump to support a physiological circulation.

CLASSIFICATION (NEW YORK HEART ASSOCIATION)[2]

I No symptoms on ordinary activity.

II Slight limitation of physical activity (comfortable at rest but ordinary activity results in fatigue and shortness of breath).

III Marked limitation of physical activity (comfortable at rest but less than ordinary activity causes symptoms).

IV Dyspnoeic at rest.

STATISTICS

➤ 1–2% of UK population have heart failure.
➤ Median age of presentation is 76 years.
➤ Prevalence increases with advancing age – less than 1% of people under 65 years are affected compared to 10–20% of the over-80s.
➤ More common in men than women (2:1).
➤ Accounts for 5% of all medical admissions.
➤ Readmission rates over a three-month period are around 50%.
➤ Number of cases is projected to rise with time.
➤ Prognosis is poor with an annual mortality rate of 10–50% depending on severity.

NATIONAL SERVICE FRAMEWORK FOR CORONARY HEART DISEASE 2000[3]
Aims

➤ To help patients with heart failure live longer and achieve better quality of life.
➤ To help patients with unresponsive heart failure receive appropriate palliative care support.

Standard

➤ Doctors should arrange for people with suspected heart failure to be offered appropriate investigations that will confirm or refute the diagnosis.
➤ For those in whom heart failure is confirmed, its cause should be identified and the treatments most likely to both relieve symptoms and reduce risk of death should be offered.

COMMON CAUSES

➤ Ischaemic heart disease.
➤ Hypertension.
➤ Valvular heart disease.
➤ Arrhythmias.
➤ Cardiomyopathies.
➤ Alcohol.
➤ Older patients can suffer acute cardiac decompensation following a non-cardiac illness, e.g. pneumonia.

DIAGNOSIS
European Society of Cardiology diagnostic criteria for chronic heart failure (2001)[4]

1 Symptoms of heart failure at rest or during exercise (dyspnoea, reduced exercise tolerance, orthopnoea, peripheral oedema).
2 Objective evidence of cardiac dysfunction.
3 Response to appropriate treatment.
➤ Older patients may not present with classic symptoms and signs, making the diagnosis challenging.
➤ Typical features, including leg swelling and shortness of breath, have a wide differential diagnosis including:

Peripheral oedema

➤ Venous insufficiency.
➤ Drug-induced fluid retention.
➤ Hypoalbuminaemia.
➤ Inactivity.
➤ Lymphoedema.

Dyspnoea

➤ Chronic obstructive airways disease.
➤ Pulmonary embolus.
➤ Anaemia.

BNP

➤ B-type natriuretic peptide.
➤ Serum level is raised in patients with heart failure. Negative predictive value of 98% makes heart failure a very unlikely diagnosis if level is low.

Other baseline tests

➤ Renal/thyroid/liver function.
➤ Full blood count.
➤ Fasting glucose and lipid profile.
➤ Urinalysis.
➤ Chest X-ray.
➤ ECG.
➤ Echocardiogram.

MANAGEMENT
Non-pharmacological

➤ Fluid and dietary salt restriction to maintain a stable weight.
➤ Regular gentle exercise as tolerated.

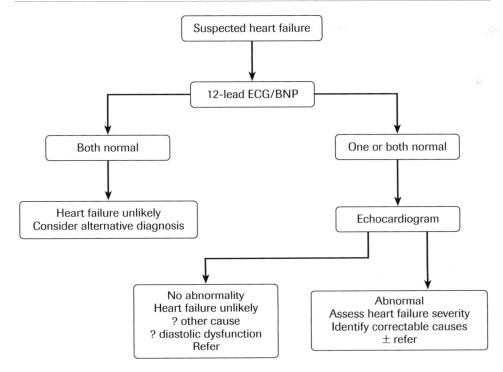

FIGURE 27.1 From NICE guidelines for diagnosis of heart failure.[1]

- ➤ Cessation of smoking.
- ➤ Limited alcohol.
- ➤ Optimisation of blood pressure control.
- ➤ Annual influenza vaccination.

Pharmacological
- ➤ Medication concordance is essential.

Diuretics
- ➤ Improve symptoms.
- ➤ No survival benefit when used alone.
- ➤ Doses can be adjusted according to requirements.
- ➤ Most patients will need a loop diuretic at some stage.
- ➤ A thiazide can be used in combination with a loop for powerful synergistic effect.
- ➤ For spironolactone see below.

Angiotensin converting enzyme inhibitors (ACE-I)
- ➤ Improve symptoms.
- ➤ Reduce mortality rate.
- ➤ Should be considered in all cases of left ventricular systolic impairment (ejection fraction <40%).
- ➤ Contraindications include severe aortic stenosis, bilateral renal artery stenosis and significant renal dysfunction.

➤ Monitor renal function (U+E before first dose, 1–2 weeks after each dose increment, then 3–6 monthly).
➤ Aim to use recommended target doses, e.g. ramipril 5 mg bd; perindopril 4 mg od.

Angiotensin II receptor antagonists
➤ Consider if ACE-I not tolerated.

β-blockers
➤ Improve survival.
➤ Consider once stable on diuretic and ACE-I.
➤ Bisoprolol and carvedilol are licensed for use in heart failure in the UK.
➤ Start at a low dose and increase slowly as tolerated over weeks/months.

Spironolactone
➤ An aldosterone antagonist potassium-sparing diuretic.
➤ Reduces mortality rate in patients with moderate/severe heart failure (New York Heart Association Classes III/IV) when combined with a conventional diuretic and ACE-I.

Digoxin
➤ For ventricular rate control in atrial fibrillation.
➤ Exerts a positive inotropic effect and so can be used for patients in sinus rhythm with severe left ventricular failure.
➤ Does not reduce mortality rate.

Vasodilators
➤ A nitrate/hydralazine combination can be used if intolerant of ACE-I/angiotensin II receptor antagonists.

Inotropes
➤ Can be considered for acutely unwell inpatients unresponsive to conventional therapy.

Other interventions in selected patients
➤ Coronary revascularisation.
➤ Cardiac resynchronisation (biventricular pacing).
➤ Implantable cardioverter defibrillators.

FOLLOW-UP
➤ Cardiology, general medical or geriatric clinics.
➤ Nurse-led heart failure monitoring service.
➤ Assessment should include:
　— symptom review
　— examination
　— weight
　— medication optimisation
　— compliance assurance
　— dietary/fluid modifications
　— renal function
　— education of patient and carer.

PROGNOSIS

➤ Worse than for some forms of cancer.
➤ Should be discussed with patients and their carers.
➤ Need to focus not just on treatments that prolong life, but on those that relieve symptoms and improve quality of life.
➤ Skills of palliative care professionals should be translated into caring for patients with severe heart failure.

DIASTOLIC HEART FAILURE

➤ Patients with symptoms of heart failure but normal left ventricular function on echocardiography.
➤ Affects 1% of the older population.
➤ Little evidence on best treatment approach.
➤ Aim to control blood pressure, relieve symptoms of fluid overload and prevent ischaemia.

REFERENCES

1 National Institute for Health and Clinical Excellence. *Chronic Heart Failure: management of chronic heart failure in adults in primary and secondary care: NICE clinical guideline 5.* London: NIHCE; 2003. Available at: www.nice.org.uk/cg5 (accessed 25 May 2010).
2 The Criteria Committee of the New York Heart Association. *Nomenclature and Criteria for Diagnosis of Diseases of the Heart and Blood Vessels.* 9th ed. Boston, MA: Little, Brown & Company; 1994; 253–6.
3 Department of Health. *National Service Framework for Coronary Heart Disease: modern standards and service models.* London: Department of Health; 2000. Available at: www.dh.gov.uk/en/Publicationsandstatistics/Publications/PublicationsPolicyAndGuidance/DH_4094275 (accessed 25 May 2010).
4 European Society of Cardiology. The taskforce for the diagnosis and treatment of chronic heart failure. *Eur Heart J.* 2001; **22**: 1527–60.

FURTHER READING

National Institute for Health and Clinical Excellence. *Cardiac Resynchronisation Therapy for the Treatment of Heart Failure. NICE technical appraisal 120.* London: NIHCE; 2007. www.nice.org.uk/TA120

CHAPTER 28

Atrial fibrillation

DEFINITION
➤ Uncoordinated electrical activity of the atria resulting in little/no effective mechanical contraction.
➤ Manifested on ECG as absence of P waves and irregular baseline of fibrillatory waves.

PATHOPHYSIOLOGY
➤ Initiated by rapid electrical discharges from atrial cells.
➤ Various trigger sites including cuffs of muscle at openings of pulmonary veins, atrial appendages and coronary sinus.
➤ Structural changes develop in atria over time (enlargement, fibrosis and hypertrophy), which perpetuate arrhythmogenesis.

CLASSIFICATION
➤ *Paroxysmal*: terminates spontaneously but recurs.
➤ *Persistent*: does not terminate spontaneously/present for <1 year.
➤ *Permanent*: cannot be terminated by either chemical or electrical cardioversion/persists for >1 year.

STATISTICS
➤ Commonest cardiac arrhythmia.
➤ Affects 0.4% total population.
➤ Prevalence increases with age:
  — <1% <60 years
  — 6–10% >80 years.
➤ Substantial risk of thromboembolic stroke:
  — risk of ischaemic stroke increased 2–7 fold in non-rheumatic cases
  — risk increases 17-fold in rheumatic atrial fibrillation (AF).

COMMON CAUSES
➤ Lone AF (no identifiable cause).
➤ Valvular heart disease, especially mitral valve.
➤ Hypertension.
➤ Ischaemic heart disease.
➤ Hyperthyroidism.
➤ Alcohol.

CLINICAL FEATURES
➤ Patients may be asymptomatic.
➤ Symptoms include palpitations, shortness of breath, fatigue, chest pain, dizziness and syncope.
➤ Cardiac ischaemia, heart failure and thromboembolic events may be precipitated.

MANAGEMENT
➤ Where possible the underlying cause should be corrected.
➤ Two important aspects to treatment:
— rate control or restoration of sinus rhythm
— prevention of thromboembolism.

Rate/rhythm control
➤ Digoxin, rate-limiting calcium channel antagonists, β-blockers and amiodarone are agents commonly used to control ventricular rate by slowing conduction through atrioventricular node.
➤ Little evidence that restoration of sinus rhythm is more favourable than rate control and anticoagulation but it may help relieve symptoms.
➤ Sinus rhythm can be regained pharmacologically (e.g. amiodarone, flecainide, propafenone) or electrically.
➤ Direct current (DC) electrical shock requires anticoagulation with international normalised ratio (INR) maintained at 2–3 for at least 3 weeks when AF has been present for >48 hours (unless transoesophageal echocardiography excludes thrombus).
➤ Long-term maintenance of sinus rhythm after DC cardioversion is poor (approximately 1/5 over 5 years).
➤ DC cardioversion success rates may be enhanced by drug prophylaxis, e.g. amiodarone, flecainide.

Prevention of thromboembolism
➤ One in six patients who has a stroke is in AF.
➤ Additional risk factors include:
— age >75
— previous stroke
— transient ischaemic attacks (TIAs)
— structural heart disease
— hypertension
— ischaemic heart disease
— left ventricular dysfunction
— diabetes mellitus.
➤ Risk of ischaemic stroke can be reduced with antiplatelet agents or anticoagulation.
➤ Aspirin at a dose of 300 mg/day decreases risk by 20%.
➤ Warfarin (optimum INR 2–3) reduces risk by 60–70%.
➤ As warfarin carries a small risk of bleeding, a risk versus benefit decision needs to be made in each case.
➤ Tight INR control reduces bleeding tendency.
➤ High-risk patients should be offered warfarin therapy assuming no contraindications preclude its use.
➤ Cautions/contraindications to warfarin include:
— recent trauma/surgery/haemorrhage
— actively bleeding gastrointestinal lesion

— uncontrolled hypertension
— falls
— alcohol misuse
— severe renal/hepatic impairment
— moderate/severe cognitive impairment
— likely non-compliance
— warfarin allergy (consider nicoumalone as an alternative).

CHADS2 scoring system:[1]

	Condition	Points
C	Congestive heart failure	1
H	Hypertension >160 mmHg or treated hypertension	1
A	Age >75	1
D	Diabetes mellitus	1
S2	Previous ischaemic stroke or TIA	2

The higher the CHADS2 score, the higher the annual stroke risk (1.9% for a score of zero/18.2% for 6 points).

Thromboprophylaxis therapy guideline:

Score	Risk	Therapy
0	Low	Aspirin 75–300 mg daily
1	Moderate	Aspirin or warfarin
≥2	High	Warfarin

➤ Older people are often inappropriately denied warfarin therapy on grounds of age alone.
➤ Decisions regarding continued warfarin use in older people should be reviewed as clinical situations may change over time, e.g. new falls.
➤ INR can be monitored in hospital anticoagulation clinics, GP surgeries or at home with the aid of district nurse services.

REFERENCE

1 Go AS *et al.* Anticoagulation therapy for stroke prevention in atrial fibrillation: how well do randomised trials translate into clinical practice? *JAMA.* 2003; **290**: 2685.

FURTHER READING

National Institute for Health and Clinical Excellence. *Atrial Fibrillation: the management of atrial fibrillation: NICE clinical guideline 36.* London: NIHCE; 2006. www.nice.org.uk/cg36

CHAPTER 29

Cardiac arrhythmias

Atrial fibrillation is the commonest arrhythmia in older people and is discussed in Chapter 28. Other arrhythmias that occur in older people are listed in Table 29.1. Bradyarrhythmias and ventricular tachycardia will be discussed in more detail here.

Bradyarrhythmias are either due to sinus node dysfunction or atrioventricular block.

SINUS NODE DYSFUNCTION

➤ The prevalence of sinus node dysfunction increases with age due to replacement of sinoatrial cells by fibrous tissue.
➤ It may manifest as sinus bradycardia, sinus arrest or brady-tachy syndrome.

Sinus bradycardia

In normal individuals, heart rates below 35–40 beats/min should not reduce cerebral perfusion sufficiently to cause symptoms. However, older patients with associated cardiovascular and cerebrovascular disease are more prone to experience symptoms such as presyncope, fatigue and dyspnoea.

Sinus pauses

Sinus pauses of <3 s are not usually associated with symptoms, whereas those ≥3 s may cause syncope or presyncope. In the absence of symptoms, it is important to be cautious in interpreting sinus arrest as a cause of syncope.

Brady-tachy syndrome/sick sinus syndrome

Patients have a combination of sinus node dysfunction causing bradycardias and atrial tachyarrhythmias (sinus/atrial tachycardia, atrial flutter or atrial fibrillation). They may present with palpitation or presyncope/syncope or a combination of both. Tachycardias often follow on bradycardias so pacemaker insertion prevents syncope and may also reduce tachyarrhythmias.

ATRIOVENTRICULAR (AV) CONDUCTION DEFECT

Heart block is a common cause of dizziness and syncope in older people. It may be transient and infrequent and therefore, difficult to demonstrate despite repeated ambulatory ECG recordings. The clinical significance depends on the site and the degree of block.

➤ *First-degree heart block.* The PR interval (>200 ms) is prolonged but 1:1 AV conduction is maintained and syncope is rare unless the PR interval is greatly prolonged (300–500 ms) causing functional AV dissociation, resulting in dizziness and hypotension.
➤ *Mobitz-type I second-degree heart block* (Wenkeback). There is progressive

TABLE 29.1 Cardiac arrhythmias in older people

Bradyarrhythmia
sinus-node dysfunction
sinus bradycardia
sinus arrest
brady-tachy syndrome
atrioventricular conduction defect
type I second degree AV block (Wenkeback)
type II second degree AV block (Mobitz II)
complete heart block

Tachyarrhythmia
supraventricular tachyarrhythmia
atrioventricular nodal node re-entrant tachycardia
atrioventricular tachycardia with WPW
atrial tachycardia
atrial flutter
atrial fibrillation
ventricular tachycardia
monomorphic ventricular tachycardia
polymorphic ventricular tachycardia
ventricular fibrillation

Arrhythmias due to pacemaker malfunction
bradycardia due to:
battery failure
generator failure
electrode dysfunction
interference (myopotential or electromagnetic)
inappropriate programming
tachycardia due to pacemaker mediated tachycardia
pacemaker syndrome

prolongation of the PR interval, followed by a blocked P wave, resulting in intermittent AV conduction. The block is usually in the AV node. It often occurs in association with high vagal tone and can be caused by drugs such as β-blockers, digoxin and calcium channel blockers. It rarely causes syncope in these circumstances. It is not usually an indication for pacing on its own but may precede the development of higher degree AV block.

➤ *Mobitz-type II second-degree AV block.* There is intermittent failure of AV conduction usually resulting in every second or third P wave being blocked. The block is usually in the His bundle or infra-His conduction tissue. Patients with type II block may have recurrent syncope and require permanent pacing.

➤ *Third-degree or complete heart block* results in complete failure of AV conduction. In older people it is usually due to degenerative disease, ischaemic heart disease or drugs. The block is usually located in the His bundle of infra-His conduction tissue and the escape rhythm may be slow and unreliable resulting in syncope. Permanent pacing is indicated even in the absence of symptoms as these patients have an increase risk of sudden death.

MANAGEMENT OF BRADYARRHYTHMIAS

➤ Exclude precipitant cause – therapy with rate-limiting drugs, such as β-blockers, digoxin, diltiazem and verapamil, and systemic problems, such as hypothyroidism and hypothermia.

➤ *Pacemaker implantation* – pacing in sinoatrial disease is indicated to improve symptoms and functional status, whereas pacing for AV block is for prognostic reasons.

➤ The terminology used to describe pacemakers applies to the chamber paced, the chamber sensed, the response to sensing, the programmable capability, and anti-tachycardia functions. The type of device inserted depends largely on the indication, and functional capacity of the individual and for most older patients will either be a single or dual chamber device with or without rate responsive mode.

➤ Cardiac resynchronisation therapy with *multi-site (biventricular) pacing* may improve symptoms in heart failure patients with NYHA class III–IV symptoms on medical therapy, QRS prolongation (>150 ms) and dyssynchronous ventricular contraction. This therapy is therefore not indicated for bradycardia but is designed to improve myocardial performance in patients with heart failure. The potential benefits of multi-site pacing in older patients with ventricular electromechanical dissociation are still uncertain but may be indicated in selected cases.

VENTRICULAR TACHYCARDIA (VT)

Sustained monomorphic VT is usually seen in patients with organic heart disease, most commonly ischaemic in nature. Ventricular fibrillation usually results in syncope and sudden death, unless the patient is defibrillated rapidly. Untreated, the recurrence rate of VT is high, especially in the presence of impaired systolic function. Treatment options depend on the underlying cause and need to be tailored to the individual. They include:

➤ treatment of ischaemia

➤ correction of electrolyte imbalance (K^+ and Mg^{2+})

➤ anti-arrhythmic drugs – β-blockers are usually first line. Amiodarone is used if they are contraindicated

➤ *Implantable cardiac defibrillator (ICDs)*. These are devices which detect abnormal ventricular rates and terminate the arrhythmia according to programmed algorithms. The ICD can terminate abnormal, fast ventricular rates by acting as an 'overdrive' pacemaker, which is known as 'anti-tachycardia pacing'. If repeated bursts of overdrive pacing fail to cardiovert VT, then an electrical shock will be administered. If VF is detected, electrical defibrillation therapy is delivered. The ICD also has pacemaker capability to deal with slow heart rates. There are now UK guidelines for the use of ICDs and while some indications are not applicable to older patients, they should be considered in those with a reasonable quality of life and prognosis.

Torsade de pointes is a type of polymorphic ventricular tachycardia, characterised by beat-to-beat variability of the amplitude and polarity of the QRS complexes. It is usually associated with prolongation of the QT interval. In older people this is usually acquired as a result of electrolyte abnormalities, drugs such as anti-arrhythmics, psychotropics and anti-microbials or hypothermia. Treatment involves elimination of the underlying cause. In the acute phase recurrences can be prevented by temporary pacing or isoprenaline infusion.

FURTHER READING

Gregoratos G, Abrams J, Epstein AE *et al.* ACC/AHA/NASPE 2002 guideline update for implantation of cardiac pacemakers and antiarrhythmia devices: summary article: a report of the American College of Cardiology American Heart Association task force on practice guidelines (ACC/AHA/NASPE Committee). *J Am Coll Cardiol.* 2002; **40**: 1703–19.

National Institute for Health and Clinical Excellence. *Implantable cardioverter defibrillators (ICDs) for the treatment of arrhythmias (review of TA11). NICE technology appraisal 95.* London: NIHCE; 2006. www.nice.org.uk/TA095

CHAPTER 30

Stroke

DEFINITION (WHO 1980)

➤ A clinical syndrome typified by rapidly developing signs of focal (at times global) disturbance of cerebral function, lasting more than 24 hours or leading to death within 24 hours, with no apparent cause other than that of vascular origin.

STATISTICS

➤ Third commonest cause of death and most frequent cause of severe disability worldwide.
➤ Incidence increases with age and is expected to rise by 20% over next 20 years as population ages.
➤ Accounts for 12% of deaths in UK.
➤ 110 000 people (2 per 1 000) have a first stroke in England and Wales each year.
➤ Past history of stroke or transient ischaemic attack (TIA) increases the risk of a further ischaemic event 13-15-fold.
➤ 30% of patients die during first month.
➤ 35% are significantly disabled at one year.
➤ 5% are admitted to long-term care.
➤ Mortality and morbidity rates are higher in the older population.
➤ Stroke care costs NHS over £2.8 billion per year.

CLASSIFICATION

➤ 85% ischaemic:
  — atherosclerotic 20%
  — penetrating artery disease 25%
  — cardiogenic embolism 20%
  — cryptogenic 30%
  — others (e.g. prothrombotic states, carotid artery dissection) 5%.
➤ Clinical syndromes depend on affected vascular territory:
  — total anterior circulation infarction (TACI) – territory supplied by middle cerebral artery (MCA)
  — partial anterior circulation infarction (PACI) – occlusion of branches of MCA or isolated anterior cerebral artery occlusion
  — posterior circulation infarction (POCI) – infarction of brainstem, cerebellum or occipital lobe
  — lacunar infarcts (LACI) – occlusion of basal perforating arteries.
➤ 15% haemorrhagic:
  — intraparenchymal
  — subarachnoid.

RISK FACTORS

➤ Age.
➤ Male gender.
➤ Afro-Caribbean and South Asian ethnic groups.
➤ Low socio-economic class.
➤ Previous stroke.
➤ History of TIA.
➤ Atrial fibrillation.
➤ Carotid artery stenosis.
➤ Valvular heart disease.
➤ Hypertension.
➤ Hypercholesterolaemia.
➤ Smoking.
➤ Diabetes mellitus.
➤ Alcohol misuse.
➤ Physical inactivity.

CONSEQUENCES OF STROKE

➤ Aspiration.
➤ Cognitive impairment.
➤ Communication difficulties.
➤ Contractures.
➤ Deep venous thrombosis.
➤ Dependency.
➤ Depression.
➤ Disability.
➤ Dysphagia.
➤ Incontinence (urinary/faecal).
➤ Infection (chest/urine).
➤ Pain (mechanical/neuropathic).
➤ Pressure sores.

PRIMARY PREVENTION

➤ Control of blood pressure.
➤ Antiplatelet/anticoagulant therapy for atrial fibrillation.
➤ Carotid endarterectomy in suitable patients.
➤ Smoking cessation.
➤ Moderate alcohol consumption.
➤ Low fat/salt intake.
➤ Exercise.

UK STROKE ASSOCIATION'S ACT FAST CAMPAIGN[1]

➤ FAST (face arm speech test) is a validated pre-hospital assessment tool that can be used to screen for stroke and TIA.
➤ Part of a major public awareness campaign.

ACUTE MANAGEMENT OF ISCHAEMIC STROKE

➤ Patients with suspected stroke should be admitted directly to a specialist acute stroke unit following initial assessment.

Antiplatelet therapy
➤ Aspirin (300 mg) is recommended as soon as possible after onset of symptoms (can be given rectally or via nasogastric tube if necessary).
➤ Can be administered to patients with suspected ischaemic stroke even when CT brain confirmation is not available (CT should be performed within 24 hours of admission).
➤ Prompt treatment reduces risk of further stroke or death in hospital and risk of death and dependency at 6 months.

Thrombolysis
➤ Alteplase (rt-PA) licensed for use in UK in patients under 80 years of age.
➤ Haemorrhage must be excluded by CT or MRI brain before administration.
➤ Improves outcome if administered to selected patients within 3 hours of acute ischaemic stroke onset by an experienced stroke physician in a specialist centre.
➤ Patients 30% more likely to have minimal/no disability 3 months post-stroke.
➤ Significantly reduces length of stay.
➤ Main complication is intracranial haemorrhage.
➤ Contraindications:
 — active internal bleeding
 — intracranial or intraspinal surgery, serious head injury or stroke within previous 3 months
 — intracranial neoplasm, arteriovenous malformation or aneurysm
 — severe uncontrolled hypertension
 — bleeding diathesis
 — warfarin with INR >1.7
 — heparin therapy with elevated activated partial thromboplastin time (APTT)
 — platelet count <100.
➤ Widespread use is limited until adequate resources allocated.

EARLY MANAGEMENT
Homeostasis
➤ Maintain adequate hydration.
➤ Control blood pressure in hypertensive emergencies.
➤ Provide supplementary oxygen if saturations <95% on air.
➤ Keep blood glucose measurements between 4 and 11 mmol/L.

Nutrition
➤ Malnutrition associated with worse outcome.
➤ Patients with an unsafe swallow should have a nasogastric tube inserted for feeding within 24 hours of admission.

Bowel and bladder
➤ Double incontinence common in severe strokes.
➤ *See* Chapter 32: Bowel and bladder management.

Positioning
➤ Important in prevention of pressure sores, contractures and pneumonia.

Deep vein thrombosis prophylaxis
➤ Ensure adequate hydration.
➤ Immobile patients should wear compression stockings if no contraindications.

➤ Subcutaneous heparin increases risk of intracerebral haemorrhage and so should not be used routinely.

REHABILITATION
Stroke units
➤ Designated stroke units offering a multidisciplinary approach to stroke care and lead by a physician with a specialist interest in stroke have been shown to reduce mortality, dependency and need for institutionalisation without prolonging length of stay.

Multidisciplinary team
➤ Physician specialising in stroke medicine.
➤ Clinical nurse specialist.
➤ Stroke care coordinator.
➤ Speech and language therapist.
➤ Physiotherapist.
➤ Occupational therapist.
➤ Dietician.
➤ Clinical psychologist.
➤ Continence advisor.
➤ Pharmacist.
➤ Social worker.
➤ Health advocates.

SECONDARY PREVENTION
➤ Risk of further stroke approximately 7% per year.
➤ Patients at highest risk in early stages.

Control of hypertension
➤ Minimum accepted blood pressure (BP) 150/90.
➤ British Hypertension Society guidelines suggest optimal BP of 140/85 (140/80 in patients with diabetes mellitus).
➤ Treatment should be commenced if BP remains elevated after one month.
➤ Combination of long-acting ACE inhibitor, e.g. ramipril or perindopril and thiazide diuretic, e.g. indapamide should be considered as first line.

Prevention of thromboembolism
➤ Patients with ischaemic stroke who are not anticoagulated should be taking antiplatelet therapy, e.g. aspirin 75 mg od, clopidogrel 75 mg od or combination of low-dose aspirin and modified-release dipyridamole 200 mg bd.
➤ Patients who have had an event whilst taking aspirin alone and in whom anticoagulation is not appropriate should be prescribed clopidogrel in addition or switched to a combination of dipyridamole modified-release and aspirin.
➤ After 14 days warfarin should be prescribed for patients in atrial fibrillation assuming haemorrhage has been excluded and no contraindications exist.
➤ Patients with carotid artery area stroke, carotid artery stenosis of 70–99% and minor/no residual disability should be considered for carotid endarterectomy, angioplasty or stent insertion (referral should be within 1 week of symptom onset and the procedure performed within 2 weeks).

ANTI-LIPID TREATMENT
➤ Statin therapy provides benefit independent of cholesterol level.

Lifestyle advice

➤ Smoking cessation.
➤ Moderate alcohol intake.
➤ Low-fat diet.
➤ Reducing salt intake.
➤ Exercise.

DISCHARGE PLANNING

➤ Close liaison between disciplines.
➤ Communication of information to GP and community services.

LONG-TERM MANAGEMENT

➤ Outpatient follow-up (further input may be required after active rehabilitation phase).
➤ Ensure maintenance of risk factor modification.
➤ Monitor for development of complications.
➤ Support for informal carers.

CARERS

➤ Informal carers need:
  — information and education about all aspects of stroke
  — to be involved in decision-making
  — emotional, financial, practical and social support
  — a named contact for advice/assistance in crises
  — details of support groups, e.g. Stroke Association
  — opportunities for respite.

TRANSIENT ISCHAEMIC ATTACK

➤ A thromboembolic event resulting in sudden onset of focal cerebral or retinal deficit that recovers within 24 hours.
➤ Duration usually less than 30 minutes.
➤ 30–40 000 people suffer TIAs in the UK each year.
➤ Source of thromboembolism most commonly carotid artery, heart, aorta or vertebrobasilar vessels.
➤ A warning sign for future stroke (15% of ischaemic strokes preceded by TIA).
➤ Risk of stroke following TIA:
  — 8–12% at 7 days
  — 11–15% at 1 month
  — 17–18% at 3 months.

ABCD2 Test – a scoring system to evaluate risk of stroke after TIA:

A	age	>60 years	1 point
B	blood pressure	≥140/90 mmHg	1 point
C	clinical features	unilateral weakness	2 points
		speech disturbance only	1 point
D	duration of symptoms	≥60 mins	2 points
		10–59 mins	1 point
2	diabetes		1 point

Low risk   0–3
Medium risk 4–5
High risk   6–7

➤ Formal assessment, modification of risk factors and initiation of preventive therapy should occur at the earliest opportunity – patients with scores of 4 and above should be managed as medical emergencies and those with scores of below 4 should be seen and investigated within 7 days.

➤ CT/MRI brain is not necessary before prescribing prophylaxis.

➤ Aspirin recommended as first line for patients in sinus rhythm (clopidogrel if aspirin-intolerant).

➤ For patients in sinus rhythm already taking aspirin, addition of a second recommended antiplatelet agent is suggested if recurrent TIAs.

➤ Warfarin is more effective than aspirin in prevention of stroke in people with atrial fibrillation (not recommended for patients in sinus rhythm).

REFERENCE

1 The Stroke Association. *Suspect a Stroke? Act FAST.* London: The Stroke Association; 2008. Available at: www.stroke.org.uk/information/recognising_stroke_with_the_fast_test/index.html (accessed 26 May 2010).

FURTHER READING

British Geriatrics Society. *Good Practice Guides: Stroke.* London: British Geriatrics Society; 2007. www.bgs.org.uk/index.php?option=com_content&view=article&id=378:stroke&catid=12:goodpractice&Itemid=106

Department of Health. *National Stroke Strategy.* London: Department of Health; 2007. www.dh.gov.uk/en/Publicationsandstatistics/Publications/PublicationsPolicyandguidance/dh_081062

Intercollegiate Stroke Working Party. *National Clinical Guidelines for Stroke.* 3rd ed. London: Royal College of Physicians; 2008. www.rcplondon.ac.uk

National Institute for Health and Clinical Excellence. *Diagnosis and Initial Management of Acute Stroke and Transient Ischaemic Attack (TIA). NICE clinical guideline 68.* London: NIHCE; 2008. www.nice.org.uk/cg68

CHAPTER 31

Movement disorders

PARKINSON'S DISEASE
Statistics
➤ One of the commonest neurological conditions affecting older people.
➤ 160 per 100 000 population are affected.
➤ Prevalence increases with age (2% of over-80s).
➤ Annual incidence 13 per 100 000.

Pathology
➤ Degeneration of dopaminergic neurones in substantia nigra.
➤ Precise aetiology unknown.
➤ Causes of parkinsonism but not true Parkinson's disease include cerebrovascular disease, drugs, e.g. neuroleptics, and Parkinson-plus disorders such as multisystem atrophy and progressive supranuclear palsy.

Clinical features
➤ Parkinson's disease has four cardinal signs:
— tremor
— rigidity
— bradykinesia
— loss of postural reflexes.

Diagnosis
United Kingdom Parkinson's Disease Society diagnostic criteria[1]
➤ Diagnosis of parkinsonism requires bradykinesia plus at least one of:
— muscular rigidity
— rest tremor
— postural instability.
➤ Exclusion criteria:
— recurrent strokes
— repeated head injuries
— encephalitis.
➤ Supportive criteria (at least three required):
— unilateral onset
— evidence of progression
— persistent asymmetry
— excellent response to L-dopa
— severe L-dopa-induced chorea
— L-dopa response for more than 5 years

— clinical course more than 10 years.

➤ Accurate diagnosis may be complicated by comorbidity, e.g. cerebrovascular disease or atypical presentation.

➤ In cases of diagnostic uncertainty a DaT (dopamine transporter) SCAN can be helpful.

Non-motor symptoms/complications
Physical
➤ Falls.

➤ Postural hypotension.

➤ Pressure sores.

➤ Urinary incontinence.

➤ Constipation.

➤ Dysphagia.

➤ Aspiration pneumonia.

➤ Dysarthria.

➤ Sleep disturbance.

Psychiatric
➤ Depression.

➤ Cognitive impairment.

➤ Hallucinations.

Social
➤ Loss of independence.

➤ Isolation.

Management
Drug therapy
➤ L-dopa commonly prescribed as a first-line agent in combination with a dopa-decarboxylase inhibitor (risk of developing motor complications over time).

➤ Dopaminergic agonists, e.g. ropinerole, pramipexole, pergolide can be used as monotherapy or as adjuncts to L-dopa (less likely to cause dyskinetic side-effects).

➤ Other therapeutic agents include monoamine-oxidase type B (MAO-B). inhibitors, e.g. selegiline, catechol-o-methyltransferase inhibitors, e.g. entacapone, and subcutaneous apomorphine in advanced disease.

➤ Rivastigmine can be of benefit in the treatment of cognitive impairment and hallucinations.

➤ Depression can be treated with selective serotonin reuptake inhibitors (SSRIs) or serotonin norepinephrine reuptake inhibitors (SNRIs) (caution with MAO-B inhibitors).

Surgery
➤ Deep-brain stimulation (STN-DBS) can improve motor symptoms in selected patients.

Multidisciplinary team involvement
➤ Care should be provided by a geriatrician with a special interest in Parkinson's disease or a neurologist in close liaison with other professionals:
    — specialist nurse
    — general practitioner
    — physiotherapist

— occupational therapist
— speech and language therapist
— psychologist
— psychiatrist
— pharmacist
— social worker
— palliative care support.

Parkinson's disease nurse specialists
➤ Offer information and support for patients and their carers.
➤ Monitor effects of medication.
➤ Anticipate potential problems.
➤ Provide continuity of care and a link between primary and secondary care services.

NICE Guidance Recommendations (2006)[2]
➤ Patient-centred care.
➤ Carer support.
➤ Information provision.
➤ Good communication.
➤ Timely untreated referral to a specialist.
➤ Regular clinical monitoring including review of non-motor symptoms.
➤ Access to specialist nursing care.
➤ Access to rehabilitation therapies.
➤ Consideration of palliative care during all phases of the disease.

ESSENTIAL TREMOR
➤ Occurs during voluntary movement.
➤ Hands and arms most commonly affected.
➤ Can affect the neck resulting in head shakes.
➤ Ability to perform activities of daily living may be affected.
➤ Symptoms worsen under stressful conditions.
➤ Beneficial effect from alcohol.
➤ Aetiology unclear.
➤ Family history often present.
➤ Increasing prevalence with age.
➤ Female predominance.
➤ Treatment options include primidone and β-blockers.

RESTLESS LEGS SYNDROME (RLS)
➤ Characterised by an urge to move the legs to relieve uncomfortable sensations such as burning or itching.
➤ Symptoms worse at rest and at night and can often disturb sleep.
➤ Involuntary periodic limb movements during sleep can also occur.
➤ Aetiology of primary RLS unclear.
➤ Secondary causes include iron deficiency and Parkinson's disease.
➤ More common with age.
➤ Symptoms more severe in older people.
➤ Dopamine agonists, opioids, benzodiazepines and anticonvulsants can be considered in the management of secondary RLS.

REFERENCES

1 Hughes AJ *et al.* Accuracy of clinical diagnosis of idiopathic Parkinson's disease: a clinico-pathological study of 100 cases. *J Neurol Neurosurg Psychiatr.* 1992; **55**: 181–4.

2 National Institute for Health and Clinical Excellence. *Parkinson's Disease: diagnosis and management in primary and secondary care. NICE clinical guideline 35.* London: NIHCE; 2006. Available at: www.nice.org.uk/cg35 (accessed 26 May 2010).

FURTHER READING

British Geriatrics Society. *Good Practice Guides: Parkinson's disease.* London: British Geriatrics Society; 2007. www.bgs.org.uk/index.php?option=com_content&view=article&id=376:parkinsonsdisease&catid=12:goodpractice&Itemid=106

Department of Health. *National Service Framework for Long-Term Neurological Conditions.* London: Department of Health; 2005. www.dh.gov.uk/en/Publicationsandstatistics/Publications/PublicationsPolicyAndGuidance/DH_4105361

CHAPTER 32

Bowel and bladder management

BOWEL
Constipation
Definition
➤ Constipation is defined as self-reporting of two or more of the following symptoms on more than 25% of occasions in the prior 3 months:
  — two or fewer bowel movements per week
  — hard stools
  — straining
  — feeling of incomplete evacuation.

Prevalence
➤ Self-reported constipation increases with age and older people with constipation primarily tend to have difficulty with rectal evacuation, straining and hard stools.
➤ Very common in immobilised older persons in whom gastrocolic reflex (peristalsis resulting from food entering the stomach) is impaired.

Causes
➤ Low dietary fibre.
➤ Dehydration.
➤ Immobility.
➤ Drugs, e.g. opiates, calcium channel blockers, diuretics, anticholinergic agents.
➤ Colorectal disease, e.g. diverticular disease, neoplasm.
➤ Metabolic conditions, e.g. hypothyroidism, diabetes mellitus, hypercalcaemia.
➤ Neurological pathology, e.g. stroke, Parkinson's disease, spinal cord injury.
➤ Depression.

Management
➤ Consider above causes and investigate where appropriate.
➤ In cases of chronic constipation:
  — increase fibre intake
  — increase fluid intake if possible
  — increase physical activity if able
  — stop constipating medications if feasible
  — stool softener, e.g. magnesium hydroxide
  — stimulant laxative, e.g. senna
  — impaction can be treated with suppositories (glycerine or bisacodyl) or enemas (microlax then phosphate) – if enemas unsuccessful proceed to manual evacuation.

Diarrhoea
Definition
➤ The passage of more than 300 mL liquid faeces in 24 hours.

Causes
➤ Constipation with overflow.
➤ Drugs, e.g. laxatives, antibiotics.
➤ Infection, e.g. viral, bacterial, parasitic.
➤ Gastrointestinal pathology, e.g. inflammatory bowel disease, malabsorption.

Management
➤ Exclude faecal impaction.
➤ Stop contributing medications if possible.
➤ Send stool specimen for analysis if appropriate (MCS, clostridium difficile, OCP).
➤ Investigate for gastrointestinal cause if clinically indicated.
➤ Rehydrate as necessary.
➤ Antidiarrhoeal agents may be required, e.g. codeine phosphate, loperamide.

Faecal incontinence
Definition
➤ Involuntary leakage of rectal contents through the anal canal.

Statistics
➤ Affects 2% of adult population.
➤ Higher prevalence in older people:
  — community dwellers up to 6%
  — residents of residential/nursing homes up to 30%.
➤ Underdetected and so undertreated.

Contributing factors
➤ Loose stool.
➤ Faecal impaction with overflow.
➤ Medication.
➤ Poor mobility (inability to reach toilet in time).
➤ Damage to anal sphincter/pelvic floor, e.g. obstetric causes especially forceps delivery, surgical procedures.
➤ Comorbidities, e.g. stroke, dementia.

Consequences
➤ Skin irritation/infection.
➤ Social isolation.
➤ Depression.
➤ Anxiety.
➤ Carer stress.
➤ Institutionalisation.

Management
➤ Increase awareness among health professionals.
➤ Investigate and treat contributing causes.
➤ Regular toileting.
➤ Adequately positioned toilet facilities.

Altered bowel habit

➤ A change in bowel habit may warrant further investigation especially in the following circumstances:
— presence of blood or mucous
— loss of appetite/weight.
➤ Lower bowel investigations to consider include barium enema, colonoscopy and CT pneumocolon – feasibility, tolerability, comorbidity and patient choice are important factors.

BLADDER
Urinary incontinence
Definition

➤ Involuntary loss of urine at least twice per week irrespective of amount lost.

Statistics

➤ More common with ageing but not a normal feature of ageing.
➤ Prevalence:
— 10–35% of community dwellers aged over 65 years
— 25–30% of older inpatients and those in residential care
— 50% of nursing home residents
— 70% of patients in continuing care
— Many symptoms are unreported.

Age-related changes in lower urinary tract

➤ Decrease in:
— bladder capacity
— ability to postpone voiding
— urinary flow rate
— urethral closing pressure.
➤ Increase in:
— post-void residual volume
— prostate size
— involuntary detrusor contractions
— nocturnal urine excretion.

Consequences

➤ Social isolation.
➤ Depression.
➤ Anxiety.
➤ Carer stress.
➤ Financial burden.
➤ Pressure sores.
➤ Rashes.
➤ Skin infections.
➤ Precipitating factor for institutionalisation.

Associated conditions

➤ Arthritis.
➤ Stroke.
➤ Parkinson's disease.
➤ Cognitive impairment.

➤ Peripheral vascular disease.
➤ Venous insufficiency.
➤ Constipation.
➤ Congestive cardiac failure.
➤ Chronic lung disease.
➤ Diabetes mellitus.

Classification

ACUTE

➤ Acronym (DIAPPERS):
   — D Delirium
   — I Infection/intercurrent illness
   — A Atrophic urethritis/vaginitis
   — P Pharmacological/drugs
   — P Psychological
   — E Excessive urine, e.g. fluid intake, diuretics, diabetes mellitus, hypercalcaemia
   — R Restricted mobility
   — S Stool impaction.

CHRONIC

1 Detrusor instability
   — commonest cause of urinary incontinence in older people regardless of gender
   — affects 10–30% of older women
   — involuntary uninhibited detrusor contractions overcome sphincter mechanisms
   — may be idiopathic, obstructive or neuropathic
   — exacerbated by anxiety or fast bladder filling, e.g. after diuretics
   — symptoms include urgency, urge incontinence, night-time incontinence, frequency (patients void repeatedly to avoid incontinence: more than seven times/24 hours) and nocturia
   — treatment options include:
      i behavioural modification:
         — aim to decrease urinary frequency to acceptable level and increase bladder volume
         — modify diet and fluid intake (avoid caffeine, 4 pints of fluid per day – fluid restriction increases bladder instability and risk of urinary tract infection)
         — ensure regular bowel habit
         — bladder retraining:
            a aim to suppress urge to void
            b time between voiding is lengthened leading to increased bladder capacity and fewer incontinent episodes
            c continue until voiding interval 3–4 hours
            d usually takes weeks or months
            e requires patient motivation and intact cognitive function
            f prompted/scheduled voiding can be used in demented patients.
      ii drugs:
         — mainstay of treatment
         — contraction of detrusor mediated by stimulation of muscarinic receptors in bladder wall by acetylcholine
         — oxybutynin has anticholinergic and direct smooth muscle relaxant properties which reduce intravesical pressure, increase bladder

capacity and decrease frequency of contraction
— side-effects (dry mouth, blurred vision, nausea, constipation) may lead to dose reduction or withdrawal
— slow-release formulation (oxybutynin-XL) is often better tolerated
— tolterodine, a muscarinic receptor antagonist with bladder selectivity and so fewer side-effects and increased compliance, is also available in long-acting XL form
— anticholinergic agents are contraindicated in narrow-angle glaucoma
— topical oestrogens for urogenital atrophy may help relieve sensation of urgency.

2 Stress incontinence
— second most common type of incontinence in older women
— urine leaks during physical activity, e.g. standing, lifting, coughing, sneezing, laughing, i.e. conditions of increased abdominal pressure
— weakness of pelvic floor and bladder neck lead to sphincter incompetence
— causes include damage during childbirth and postmenopausal atrophy due to oestrogen deficiency
— men may develop post-prostatectomy stress incontinence due to iatrogenic sphincter damage
— treatment methods include:
  a pelvic floor exercises:
    — aim to improve tone of pelvic floor muscles especially levator ani
    — vaginal examination essential to ensure ablility to contract correct muscle before exercises are taught
    — continence may take more than 3 months
  b biofeedback with a vaginal or rectal sensor can be used to monitor results of patient effort
  c electrical stimulation helps pelvic floor develop new fibres
  d hormone replacement therapy – urethra and trigone of bladder are sensitive to oestrogen
  e surgery can be considered in some cases (comorbidity may preclude this).

3 Retention and overflow
— large post-void residual volume
— continuous dribbling incontinence results
— recurrent urinary tract infections common
— constipation and anticholinergic drugs exacerbate symptoms
— causes include outflow tract obstruction, diabetes mellitus, injury to nerves supplying bladder
— detrusor underactivity unlikely to be the main problem.

4 Outflow obstruction
— almost always in men
— symptoms include hesitancy, poor urinary stream, post-micturition dribbling and feeling of inadequate emptying
— in chronic outflow obstruction detrusor may be replaced with fibrosis so bladder fails to empty even when obstruction is removed
— causes include benign prostatic hypertrophy (BPH), prostate cancer and urethral stricture
— one in three men referred for prostatectomy because of obstructive symptoms have an overactive detrusor for which surgery is not appropriate
— BPH:
  i prevalence rises with age (50% of men aged 50–60 and 90% of those aged over 85 years)

    ii symptoms:
- irritative: urgency, frequency, nocturia, urge incontinence
- obstructive: hesitancy, straining, feeling of incomplete emptying, retention, overflow incontinence, poor stream

    iii investigations: history, urinary symptoms review, rectal examination, urinalysis, renal function, PSA

    iv refer to urologist if:
- moderate to severe symptoms
- history of recurrent urinary tract infections
- suspicious prostate
- PSA more than 4
- palpable bladder
- failure to respond to medical treatment

    v treatment depends on symptom severity and comorbidity

    vi medical treatments:
- α-blockers, e.g. alfuzosin, doxazosin, tamsulosin
- 5 α-reductase inhibitors, e.g. finasteride

    vii side-effects of TURP:
- 70% retrograde ejaculation
- 14% impotence
- urinary incontinence in up to 15%.

5 Functional
- due to inability to reach and use toilet in time
- associated with poor mobility, loss of manual dexterity, confusion, communication problems and reduced motivation, e.g. depression.

6 Neurogenic
- damage to neuronal control of bladder function
- different lesions cause different effects:
  - loss of voluntary inhibition causes frequency, urgency, incontinence (stroke, frontal lobe tumour)
  - atonic bladder leads to retention and overflow
  - spinal cord damage results in reflex voiding
  - local irritation, e.g. bladder stone or tumour causes sensory urgency ± incontinence.

7 Mixed
- combined urge and stress incontinence is common in older women.

NATIONAL SERVICE FRAMEWORK FOR OLDER PEOPLE (STANDARD 3): PATIENT-CENTRED CARE (2001)[2]
Integrated continence services
Aims
➤ To support older people and their carers.
➤ To be in line with published guidance on good practice.
➤ To link identification (community dwellers/care home residents/hospital inpatients), assessment and treatment across primary care and acute/specialist care.
➤ To provide links to designated specialities, e.g. urology and regional/national units for specialist surgery.
➤ To provide continence aids/equipment.
➤ To provide access to bathing and laundry services.

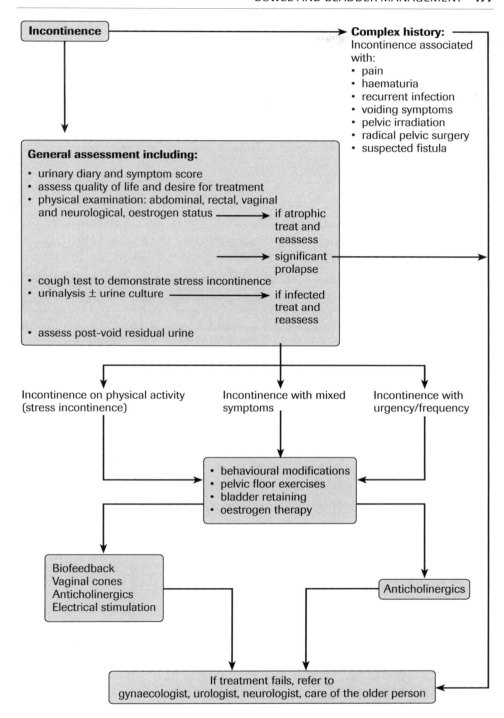

FIGURE 32.1 Incontinence treatment pathway.[1]

BRITISH GERIATRICS SOCIETY: *A GUIDE FOR THOSE WORKING IN RESIDENTIAL AND NURSING HOMES* (1998)[3]

Rationale

➤ Urinary incontinence should not be seen as inevitable.
➤ Many cases may be preventable.
➤ Good management should make untreatable cases more acceptable.

Assessment

➤ Establish patient's and carer's views of the problem and the impact it has on quality of life.
➤ Complete fluid balance and voiding charts.
➤ Ensure regular bowel action.

Management

➤ Ensure care home staff are trained in continence promotion.
➤ Provide assisted toileting for those with mobility/dexterity problems.
➤ Enlist assistance of GP to identify conditions that may exacerbate symptoms and treat as appropriate, e.g. infection, oestrogen deficiency, diabetes mellitus.
➤ Refer to continence nurse specialist for advice if required.
➤ Review medication and discontinue unnecessary drugs, e.g. diuretics, sedatives.
➤ Toileting regimes:
  — aim to ensure bladder emptying before incontinence occurs
  — optimum time between visits should be determined by voiding record.
➤ Continence pads:
  — available through community nursing or social services
  — various sizes and absorbencies
  — heavier pads for night-time use
  — mesh pants to keep in position
  — may lead to dependence and acceptance that incontinence is expected and irreversible.
➤ Sheaths:
  — need to ensure correct size
  — may cause local skin irritation and infection.
➤ Catheters:
  — intermittent catheterisation (self or staff) may be an option
  — long-term indwelling catheter may be required, e.g. persistent retention, non-healing pressure sores, to promote comfort
  — available on prescription
  — need to be changed every 6 weeks to prevent blockage
  — increase risk of infection
  — all have bacteriuria – only treat if symptomatic
  — may use leg bag or open valve at intervals.

DEPARTMENT OF HEALTH: *GOOD PRACTICE IN CONTINENCE SERVICES* (2000)[4]

➤ Integrated services.
➤ Clinical audit.
➤ Identify conditions that may exacerbate incontinence, e.g. chronic cough.
➤ Staff training.
➤ General advice to patients and carers, e.g. diet/fluid intake.
➤ Bladder training.
➤ Pelvic floor and anal sphincter exercises.

➤ Review medication, e.g. diuretics.
➤ Manage faecal impaction.
➤ Measure changes in urinary symptoms from before treatment to 6 months later.
➤ Measure patient satisfaction 6 months after treatment.
➤ Issue continence aids only after an initial assessment and/or a management/treatment plan has been completed (prematurely can lead to psychological dependence and reluctance to attempt curative treatment).
➤ Improve staff knowledge about products, e.g. handheld urinals for women.

URINARY TRACT INFECTION
Definition
➤ An infection affecting any part of the urinary tract.

Statistics
➤ A common problem in the older population.
➤ Female to male ratio is 2:1.

Symptoms and signs
➤ May be asymptomatic.
➤ Non-specific, e.g. lethargy, confusion, falls.
➤ Dysuria.
➤ Frequency.
➤ Urgency.
➤ Incontinence.
➤ Suprapubic pain.
➤ Fever.
➤ Haematuria.

Predisposing factors
➤ Anatomical or physiological abnormalities of the genitourinary tract, e.g. prostatic enlargement, strictures and stones.
➤ Indwelling urinary catheters.
➤ Diabetes mellitus.
➤ Medications, e.g. steroids.

Diagnosis
➤ Presence of nitrites/leucocytes on urinalysis is suggestive.
➤ Urine culture (mid-stream, in/out catheter) or catheter specimen if indwelling system.

Organisms
➤ *Escherichia coli* is most common.
➤ Others include proteus, klebsiella and enterococcus.

Treatment
➤ Antibiotics should be prescribed in accordance with local policy.
➤ A 3-day course of treatment should suffice in uncomplicated infections in women.
➤ Complicated infections in women and infections in men should be treated for 7 days.

Complications
➤ Delirium.
➤ Septicaemia.
➤ Renal failure.

Recurrent urinary tract infections
➤ Consider further investigations, e.g. ultrasound of renal tract, intravenous urogram.
➤ Prophylactic antibiotics may be required in some cases.

Asymptomatic bacteriuria
➤ Common in older people.
➤ Does not require antibiotic treatment.

OTHER URINARY COMPLAINTS
Nocturia
➤ Greater than twice per night.
➤ Disrupts sleeping pattern.
➤ Older people pass more urine at night (redistribution of fluid, e.g. peripheral oedema, reduced renal concentrating ability and increased GFR in supine position).
➤ Careful timing of caffeine, alcohol and certain medications is required.

Polyuria
➤ Treat possible contributing causes, e.g. diabetes mellitus, hypercalcaemia, diabetes insipidus.

REFERENCES
1 Abrams P, Khoury S, Wein A. *Incontinence Abstracts from Proceedings of the 1st International Consultation on Incontinence*. London: Health Publications; 1999.
2 Department of Health. *National Service Framework for Older People*. London: Department of Health; 2001. Available at: www.dh.gov.uk/en/publicationsandstatistics/publications/publicationspolicyandguidance/dh_4003066 (accessed 26 May 2010).
3 British Geriatrics Society. *Continence Care: a guide for those working in residential and nursing homes. Compendium document B2*. London: British Geriatrics Society; 1998. Available at: www.bgs.org.uk/Publications/Reference%20Material/reference_material_index.htm#incontinence (accessed 26 May 2010).
4 Department of Health. *Good Practice in Incontinence Services*. London: Department of Health; 2000. Available at: www.dh.gov.uk/en/Publicationsandstatistics/Publications/PublicationsPolicyAndGuidance/DH_4005851 (accessed 26 May 2010).

FURTHER READING
British Geriatrics Society. *Faecal Incontinence and Constipation in the Older Person*. London: British Geriatrics Society; 2002. www.bgs.org.uk/index.php?option=com_content&view=article&id=241:faecalincontinence&catid=8:incontinence&Itemid=258
British Geriatrics Society. *Good Practice Guides: Continence*. London: British Geriatrics Society; 2007. www.bgs.org.uk/index.php?option=com_content&view=article&id=377:continence&catid=12:goodpractice&Itemid=106
National Institute for Health and Clinical Excellence. *Urinary Incontinence: the management of urinary incontinence in women. NICE clinical guideline 40*. London: NIHCE; 2006. www.nice.org.uk/cg40
National Institute for Health and Clinical Excellence. *Faecal Incontinence: the management of faecal incontinence in adults. NICE clinical guideline 49*. London: NIHCE; 2007. www.nice.org.uk/cg49

CHAPTER 33

Gastro-oesophageal reflux disease

DEFINITION
➤ Gastro-oesophageal reflux disease is a backflow of gastric contents into the oesophagus resulting in oesophageal damage and/or a negative impact on quality of life as a result of dyspeptic symptoms.

AETIOLOGY
➤ Prevalence of reflux-related symptoms rises with age (more than 20% of over-65s).
➤ Contributing factors include:
— age-related changes in upper gastrointestinal tract
— medication (especially NSAIDs)
— difficulty maintaining an upright posture after eating.

CLINICAL FEATURES
➤ Heartburn (retrosternal/epigastric burning).
➤ Postprandial epigastric pain.
➤ Nocturnal symptoms may be associated with poor sleep and respiratory problems secondary to aspiration.
➤ Alarm features indicating the need for specialist referral for consideration of endoscopy include:[1]
— dysphagia/odynophagia
— persistent vomiting
— unexplained weight loss
— iron deficiency anaemia
— epigastric mass
— aged 55 or older with unexplained and persistent recent-onset dyspepsia alone.

LONG-TERM CONSEQUENCES
➤ Barrett's oesophagus and oesophageal cancer.
➤ Oesophageal stricture/ulceration.
➤ Chronic cough.

DIAGNOSIS
➤ May be complicated by:
— atypical symptoms
— comorbidity, e.g. ischaemic heart disease.
➤ Proton pump inhibitor (PPI) trial if no alarm features.

TREATMENT

➤ General advice:
  — avoid large meals
  — avoid lying down after eating
  — lose weight if overweight
  — stop smoking
  — reduce alcohol intake
  — elevate head of bed.
➤ Discontinue contributing medication if possible (otherwise continue with PPI prophylaxis).
➤ PPIs are the treatment of choice.
➤ NICE guidelines for PPI use in dyspepsia:
  i mild dyspepsia:
    • antacids, alginates or H2 receptor antagonists before PPI.
  ii severe dyspepsia:
    • healing dose PPI until symptoms controlled then lowest dose to maintain control
    • restart at higher dose if recurrent symptoms.

REFERENCE

1 National Institute for Health and Clinical Excellence. *Dyspepsia: management of dyspepsia in adults in primary care. NICE clinical guideline 17*. London: NIHCE; 2004. Available at: www.nice.org.uk/cg17 (accessed 26 May 2010).

CHAPTER 34

Chronic obstructive pulmonary disease

DEFINITION
➤ A disorder characterised by airflow obstruction, which is usually progressive, not fully reversible and does not change markedly over several months.
➤ Airflow obstruction is defined as reduced FEV_1 (forced expiratory volume in 1 second) and a reduced FEV_1/FVC (forced vital capacity) ratio such that FEV_1 <80% predicted and FEV_1/FVC <0.7.

PATHOLOGY
➤ Chronic inflammation, most commonly secondary to tobacco smoke, leads to damage of the airways and lung parenchyma.

STATISTICS
➤ Results in 30 000 deaths in UK each year (sixth most common cause of death).
➤ A major cause of mortality and morbidity in older people.
➤ 1% of UK population have COPD (incidence rises steeply with age).
➤ Exerts considerable economic burden on NHS (£500 million/year).
➤ 16% of medical hospital admissions are for COPD.
➤ Average length of inpatient stay is 10 days.
➤ Responsible for majority of pressure during winter bed crises.

DIAGNOSIS
➤ Underdetected and misdiagnosed.
➤ No single diagnostic test.
➤ Diagnosis should be based on a combination of:
  — symptoms
  — signs
  — spirometry (assessment of airway obstruction)

	FEV_1% predicted
mild	50–80%
moderate	30–49%
severe	<30%

➤ Treatment options include:
  — controlled oxygen therapy
  — bronchodilators
  — oral steroids
  — antibiotics
  — ventilatory support (non-invasive and invasive).

➤ Exacerbations typically present with worsening dyspnoea, wheeze, chest tightness and productive cough (note change in sputum colour, consistency and volume).

➤ Early recognition of an exacerbation is vital.

MANAGEMENT

➤ Multidisciplinary approach to care (including physiotherapy, occupational therapy, social services, dietetics and palliative care in end-stage disease).

➤ Smoking cessation should be encouraged at any age.

➤ Use of nicotine replacement products increases long-term abstinence.

➤ Short-acting inhaled bronchodilators are mainstay of symptomatic treatment (β2-agonist, e.g. salbutamol or anticholinergic agent, e.g. ipratropium bromide).

➤ Long-acting inhaled bronchodilators (β2-agonist, e.g. salmeterol or anticholinergic, e.g. tiotropium) should be added if still symptomatic on short-acting preparations or if ≥2 exacerbations per year.

➤ Inhaled corticosteroids should be considered in patients with an FEV_1 ≤50% predicted and who have had ≥2 exacerbations requiring treatment with antibiotics and/or oral steroids within 12 months.

➤ Ability to use an inhaler should be tested prior to initiating inhaled therapy and technique reviewed regularly.

➤ Spacer devices are available to ease administration of inhaled products.

➤ Nebulised bronchodilators will be required if disabling symptoms persist despite maximum inhaled treatment.

➤ Maintenance oral steroids may be required in advanced cases (remember osteoporosis prophylaxis).

➤ Theophyllines should only be prescribed after trials of short- and long-acting inhaled bronchodilators.

➤ Consider mucolytic agents in chronic productive cough.

➤ Treat oedema of cor pulmonale with diuretics.

➤ Long-term oxygen is indicated for patients with a pO_2 <7.3 kPa when stable or 7.3–8 kPa when stable and one of the following is present: polycythaemia, nocturnal hypoxaemia, peripheral oedema or pulmonary hypertension.

➤ Offer annual influenza vaccination and pneumococcal vaccination.

➤ Consider antiviral agents (zanamivir, oseltamivir) for at-risk patients presenting within 48 hours of onset of influenza-like symptoms.

➤ Stress importance of responding promptly to symptoms of an exacerbation (including medication self-management).

➤ Treat anxiety and depression.

➤ NICE (2004)[1] recommends that patients who consider themselves to be functionally disabled by COPD should be offered pulmonary rehabilitation:
  — contraindications include immobility, unstable angina and recent myocardial infarction
  — programme should be tailored to individual needs
  — interventions include physical training, education, nutritional advice and assessment of psychological/social needs.

➤ Development of respiratory assessment services will place greater emphasis on:
  — community-based care, e.g. Hospital at Home for suitable patients hence avoiding the emergency department
  — discharge from hospital, e.g. Respiratory Early Discharge Service to shorten length of stay and reduce risk of developing hospital acquired infections.

EXACERBATIONS

➤ An exacerbation is a sustained worsening of symptoms that begins acutely.
➤ They contribute to decline of lung function and progression of disease over time.
➤ 'Frequent exacerbators' are more likely to be housebound because of reduced exercise tolerance, have an increased risk of being admitted to hospital and have a poor prognosis.

TABLE 34.1 Factors to consider when deciding where to manage a patient with an exacerbation of COPD[1]

Factor	Favours hospital treatment	Favours home treatment
Able to manage at home	No	Yes
Breathlessness	Severe	Mild
General condition	Poor/deteriorating	Good
Level of activity	Poor/confined to bed	Good
Cyanosis	Yes	No
Worsening peripheral oedema	Yes	No
Level of consciousness	Impaired	Normal
Already receiving LTOT	Yes	No
Social circumstances	Living alone/not coping	Good
Acute confusion	Yes	No
Rapid rate of onset	Yes	No
Significant comorbidity	Yes	No
SaO_2 <90%	Yes	No
Chest X-ray changes	Yes	No
Arterial pH level	<7.35	≥7.35
Arterial pO_2	<7 kPa	≥7 kPa

REFERENCE

1 National Institute for Health and Clinical Excellence. *Chronic Obstructive Pulmonary Disease: the management of chronic obstructive pulmonary disease in adults in primary and secondary care. NICE clinical guideline 12*. London: NIHCE; 2004. Available at: www.nice.org.uk/cg12 (accessed 26 May 2010).

CHAPTER 35

Community-acquired pneumonia

DEFINITION OF PNEUMONIA
➤ Symptoms of an acute lower respiratory tract infection, including a cough and at least one other lower respiratory tract symptom, plus at least one systemic symptom and new focal chest signs on examination.

STATISTICS
➤ A major cause of mortality and morbidity in older people.
➤ Responsible for 10% of all deaths in the UK each year.
➤ 70% of patients admitted to hospital with community-acquired pneumonia are aged over 75.

DIAGNOSIS
➤ Challenging in the older population.
➤ Clinical features may be atypical and non-specific, e.g. confusion.
➤ Fever may be absent.
➤ Microscopy and culture of sputum may yield the causative organism but antibiotic treatment should not be delayed.
➤ Consider pulmonary tuberculosis if persistent productive cough, systemic symptoms or high-risk group (ethnic background, social deprivation).

SEVERITY ASSESSMENT
➤ In conjunction with clinical judgement the British Thoracic Society recommends use of the 5-point CURB-65 score:[1]
  — **C**onfusion (new/mental test score ≤8)
  — **U**rea (>7 mmol/L)
  — **R**espiratory rate (≥30/minute)
  — **B**lood pressure (systolic <90 mmHg and/or diastolic ≤60 mmHg)
  — age ≥65 years
  — 0–1 low risk of death (<5%)
  — 2 moderate risk of death (9%)
  — ≥3 high risk of death (15–40%)
  — patients scoring ≥2 should be referred to hospital for assessment.

Other markers of poor prognosis
➤ Significant comorbidity, e.g. renal/heart failure.
➤ Hypoxaemia (O_2 saturations <90%/pO_2 <8 kPa).
➤ Bilateral or multilobar involvement on chest film.

MANAGEMENT

➤ Most common organisms in older people are *Streptococcus pneumoniae*, *Haemophilus influenzae* and the influenza viruses.

➤ Chlamydia pneumonia may be important in residents of care homes.

➤ Place of management (home or hospital) depends on severity of episode.

➤ General measures include rest, smoking cessation, maintenance of hydration and simple analgesia for pleuritic chest pain.

➤ Early treatment with antibiotics in suitable patients shortens duration of illness and reduces mortality risk.

➤ For low severity cases managed in the community the British Thoracic Society guidelines[2] suggest oral amoxicillin 500 mg tds (or doxycycline 200 mg loading then 100 mg od or clarithromycin 500 mg bd if penicillin allergic) for 7 days.

➤ Patients (and/or carers) should be educated about when to seek help if managed at home – these cases require early medical review.

➤ Influenza and pneumococcal immunisations are recommended for everyone over the age of 65 years.

REFERENCES

1 Lim WS *et al.* Defining community-acquired pneumonia severity on presentation to hospital: an international derivation and validation study. *Thorax.* 2003; **58**: 377–82.

2 British Thoracic Society. *Guidelines for the Management of Community-acquired Pneumonia in Adults.* London: British Thoracic Society; 2009. Available at: www.brit-thoracic.org.uk/clinicalinformation/pneumonia/pneumoniaguidelines.aspx (accessed 26 May 2010).

CHAPTER 36

Diabetes mellitus

DEFINITION

➤ Diabetes mellitus is a chronic, progressive disease characterised by a raised blood glucose level.

PATHOLOGY

➤ Type I: insulin insufficiency results from autoimmune destruction of insulin-secreting pancreatic β-cells.
➤ Type II: results from defects in insulin secretion or insulin insensitivity.

STATISTICS

➤ Affects more than 2 million of the UK population (Type I 15%, Type II 85%).
➤ One of the most common chronic diseases affecting older people.
➤ Incidence is increasing in all age groups (projected rise of more than 40% by 2023).
➤ Prevalence rises with age (over 65 years: 1 in 20; over 85 years: 1 in 5).
➤ High rates of hospitalisation with long lengths of stay.
➤ An independent risk factor for admission to a care home.
➤ Most older people have Type II diabetes.
➤ More common in certain ethnic groups (South Asian, African, Afro-Caribbean and Middle Eastern).
➤ Diabetes care is costly – £4.9 billion/year (9% of total NHS budget).

DIAGNOSIS

➤ Diabetes:
  — random plasma glucose >11.1 mmol/L
  — fasting plasma glucose >7 mmol/L
  — 2-hour post-prandial glucose >11.1 mmol/L.
➤ Impaired glucose tolerance:
  — 2-hour post-glucose load 7.8–11.1 mmol/L.
➤ Impaired fasting glucose:
  — fasting plasma glucose 6.1–6.9 mmol/L.
➤ Normal:
  — fasting plasma glucose <6.1 mmol/L
  — 2-hour post-prandial glucose <7.8 mmol/L.

COMPLICATIONS

➤ Life expectancy is reduced by more than 20 years in Type I and up to 10 years in Type II.

➤ Cardiovascular disease is the most common cause of death (coronary heart disease mortality is five times higher and stroke mortality three times higher than in the non-diabetic population).
➤ Poor glycaemic control increases the risk of long-term consequences.
➤ United Kingdom Prospective Diabetes Study (UKPDS) 1998:[1] effective control of blood glucose and blood pressure can reduce/delay onset of complications.
➤ Microvascular complications:
  — retinopathy:
    i   visual impairment
    ii blindness.
  — nephropathy: renal failure (microalbuminuria of >30 mg/L is an early indicator of renal involvement/proteinuria of >300 mg/day occurs in progressive disease).
  — neuropathy:
    i   loss of sensation (predisposition to foot ulcers)
    ii   postural hypotension
    iii impotence
    iv   urinary retention
    v   diarrhoea.
➤ Macrovascular complications:
  — cardiovascular:
    i   ischaemic heart disease
    ii heart failure.
  — cerebrovascular:
    i   stroke
    ii transient ischaemic attack.
  — peripheral: amputation.
➤ Other complications:
  — cataracts
  — infections (skin/urine)
  — loss of functional independence
  — depression.

TREATMENT OF TYPE II DIABETES
➤ Dietary regulation.
➤ Increased physical activity.
➤ Patient/carer education.
➤ Control of hypertension.
➤ Control of hyperlipidaemia.
➤ Smoking cessation.
➤ Secondary prevention measures for ischaemic heart disease (aspirin, β-blockers).
➤ ACE inhibition for microalbuminuria.
➤ Regular foot care.
➤ Annual review (dilated eye examination, sensory testing, palpation of peripheral pulses).
➤ Individual care plan (home monitoring with district nurse support if required, realistic glycaemic goals).
➤ Minimise hypoglycaemia and adverse drug events.

Oral treatment
➤ Biguanides (e.g. metformin):
    i   lower blood glucose primarily by reducing hepatic gluconeogenesis

    ii   often used in overweight patients as weight loss may be a side-effect

    iii may cause lactic acidosis

    iv should be avoided in renal impairment

    v   gastrointestinal side-effects such as anorexia, nausea and diarrhoea may preclude use.

➤ Sulphonylureas (e.g. gliclazide, glipizide):

    i   increase pancreatic β-cell secretion of insulin

    ii   often used first line in non-overweight patients

    iii shorter-acting preparations preferred (avoid glibenclamide in view of long half-life).

➤ A-glucosidase inhibitors (e.g. acarbose):

    i   inhibit conversion of non-absorbable starch and sucrose into absorbable monosaccharides such as glucose

    ii   reduce rate of glucose uptake into bloodstream and lower post-prandial blood glucose levels

    iii modest effects only

    iv side-effects include abdominal bloating, flatulence and diarrhoea.

➤ Thiazolidinediones (e.g. pioglitazone, rosiglitazone):

    i   reduce peripheral and hepatic insulin resistance and decrease glucose levels by augmenting insulin-mediated peripheral glucose disposal

    ii   used as a combination treatment in patients with insufficient glycaemic control despite maximum tolerated doses of either metformin or sulphonylurea

    iii avoid in cardiac/renal/hepatic failure

    iv caution in patients at risk of fracture.

➤ DPP-4 inhibitors (e.g. sitagliptin, vildagliptin):

    i   block dipeptidyl peptidase-4

    ii   increase incretin levels which inhibit glucagon release and stimulate insulin secretion.

➤ Exenatide:

    i   a glucagon-like peptide-1 mimetic

    ii   stimulates insulin release

    iii used in obese patients.

➤ Metaglinides (e.g. repaglinide, nateglinide):

    i   stimulate release of insulin from pancreatic β-cells

    ii   similar to sulphonylureas but act at separate sites

    iii short duration and fast action mean post-prandial glucose spikes are reduced

    iv can be used as monotherapy or with metformin

    v   avoid in hepatic impairment

    vi notable drug interactions: diuretics, ACE inhibitors, salicylates, α-blockers and statins.

➤ Insulin:

    i   required in Type I diabetes

    ii   approximately 40% of patients with Type II diabetes will eventually need insulin

    iii indicated if poor glycaemic control with symptoms/persistently raised HbA1c >9%/persistent ketonuria despite dietary regulation and maximal oral therapy, continuing weight loss, severe intercurrent illness, hyperosmolar non-ketotic coma (HONK) and in specific situations, e.g. post-myocardial infarction

    iv aim is to simulate normal insulin secretion in response to dietary intake, exercise levels and metabolic state

    v   various regimens available:

    a   glargine, a long-acting insulin analogue with more predictable glycaemic control, is recommended by NICE for patients with frequent hypoglycaemic episodes, for those who require assistance from a carer or health professional to administer injections and for patients who would otherwise need twice-daily injections plus oral therapy

    b   pre-loaded pen devices simplify administration

    c   assistance of carers or district nurses may be required.

NICE GUIDELINES FOR TREATMENT OF TYPE II DIABETES[2]

➤ Individual needs and preferences should be taken into account.

➤ Good communication and education are essential.

➤ Lifestyle advice on diet and physical activity should be first-line approaches.

➤ Metformin is first line in terms of drug therapy.

➤ Second-line agents include sulphonylureas, thiazolidinediones and DPP-4 inhibitors.

➤ Third-line combinations include first- and second-line agents, exenatide and insulin.

HOME MONITORING OF GLYCAEMIC CONTROL

➤ Complicated by comorbidity, e.g. poor eyesight, arthritis, cognitive impairment.

➤ Urine dipstick monitoring pre-prandially once a week is often sufficient for patients with diet- or tablet-controlled Type II diabetes.

➤ Blood glucose monitoring recommended for patients with Type I and those with Type II on insulin.

➤ Twice-daily BMs if poor control or 4-point profile once weekly if stable.

➤ Fasting measurements of 7–9 mmol/L and random readings of 8–11 mmol/L should be sufficient to avoid hypo- and hyperglycaemic episodes.

➤ Tight control may not always be possible in older people:
— risk of hypoglycaemia
— intolerance of medication
— polypharmacy/drug interactions.

➤ Hypoglycaemia:
— predisposing factors include:
    i   poor/erratic nutritional intake
    ii impaired perception or response to hypoglycaemia secondary to cognitive difficulties
    iii dependence or isolation limiting early treatment
    iv comorbidity leading to misdiagnosis
    v impaired renal/hepatic metabolism.

DIABETES IN CARE HOMES

➤ 10% of care home residents have diabetes.

➤ A particularly vulnerable group.

➤ British Diabetic Association recommendations:[3]
— screening on entry to care facility and then every 2 years
— individualised diabetes care and dietary plans for all residents with known diabetes
— support to enable residents to manage their diabetes where this is feasible
— avoidance of unnecessary and inappropriate medical interventions
— annual review (preferably in care home) including history, examination, review of glycaemic control and medication, dilated fundoscopy, assessment of visual acuity and renal function

— access to health professionals including doctor, diabetes specialist nurse, dietician, podiatrist and optician

— educational training programme for care home staff.

NATIONAL SERVICE FRAMEWORK FOR DIABETES[4]
Relevant standards

➤ Prevention of Type II diabetes.
➤ Identification of people with diabetes.
➤ Empowering people with diabetes.
➤ Clinical care of adults with diabetes.
➤ Management of diabetic emergencies.
➤ Care of people with diabetes during admission to hospital.
➤ Detection and management of long-term complications.

REFERENCES

1 UK Prospective Diabetes Study Group. Tight blood pressure control and risk of macrovascular and microvascular complications in Type 2 Diabetes–UK PDS 38. *BMJ.* 1998; **317**: 703–13.

2 National Institute for Health and Clinical Excellence. *Type 2 Diabetes: newer agents (partial update of CG66). NICE clinical guideline 87.* London: NIHCE; 2009. Available at: www.nice. org.uk/cg87 (accessed 25 May 2010).

3 Guidelines and Practice for Residents with Diabetes in Care Homes. *A Report prepared by a Working Party of the British Diabetic Association.* London: Diabetes Care Advisory Committee; 1999.

4 Department of Health. *National Service Framework for Diabetes.* London: Department of Health; 2001. Available at: www.dh.gov.uk/en/Publicationsandstatistics/Publications/ PublicationsPolicyAndGuidance/DH_4002951 (accessed 25 May 2010).

CHAPTER 37

Renal disease

ACUTE KIDNEY INJURY
Definition
➤ A sudden decline in renal function over hours/days as evidenced by a rise in serum creatinine and a decline in glomerular filtration.
➤ Can occur in people with previously normal renal function or in those with background chronic kidney disease.

Statistics
➤ Increasingly common, especially in the older population.
➤ 1% of general hospital admissions are due to acute renal impairment.
➤ Implicated in 7% of inpatient episodes.
➤ Rates are higher for patients in intensive care settings.
➤ People with pre-existing renal dysfunction, diabetes mellitus, hypertension and vascular disease are at particularly high risk.
➤ Mortality rates can reach 75%.
➤ Prognosis is poorer in older people and those with significant comorbid conditions.

Causes
➤ Traditionally categorised into three groups:
  — pre-renal
    i   due to renal hypoperfusion
    ii   contributing factors include volume depletion, reduced cardiac output, systemic vasodilation and drugs such as diuretics and NSAIDs.
  — renal
    i   intrinsic renal damage
    ii   acute tubular necrosis is the most common cause, usually occurring secondary to an ischaemic, toxic (e.g. aminoglycosides, myoglobin deposition) or septic insult
    iii other disorders including acute glomerulonephritis and acute interstitial nephritis may be responsible.
  — post-renal
    i   a common cause of acute renal failure in older people
    ii   results from urinary tract obstruction, e.g. benign prostatic hypertrophy, carcinoma of the prostate
    iii often reversible if the obstruction is relieved early.
➤ Often multifactorial.

Assessment

➤ History
  — detailed medical and drug history (including details of over-the-counter medications) is required.
➤ Examination
  — assessment of fluid status is vital.
➤ Urinalysis
  — exclude infection
  — detect proteinuria/haematuria.
➤ Renal ultrasound scan
  — exclude obstruction
  — assess renal size.
➤ Renal biopsy
  — may be required in some cases.

Management

➤ Initiate treatment for hyperkalaemia, metabolic acidosis and pulmonary oedema if applicable.
➤ Optimise fluid status.
➤ Identify and treat precipitating cause/s.
➤ Discontinue nephrotoxic drugs.
➤ Avoid administration of any new potentially nephrotoxic agents.
➤ Adjust drug doses in accordance with glomerular filtration rate.
➤ Remember nutritional support.
➤ Liaise with nephrology and intensive care at an early stage.
➤ Indications for dialysis in acute kidney injury include:
  — refractory hyperkalaemia
  — unresolving acidosis
  — intractable fluid overload
  — symptomatic uraemia.

CHRONIC KIDNEY DISEASE
Definition

➤ A reduced glomerular filtration rate and/or kidney damage (proteinuria, haematuria or structural disease) for more than 3 months.

Statistics

➤ 1 in 10 people has some degree of chronic renal impairment.
➤ High prevalence among the older population.
➤ 50% of those over 75 years are affected.
➤ More common in black and ethnic minority groups.
➤ Many die from cardiovascular disease before reaching end-stage disease.
➤ 2% of the NHS budget is spent on renal replacement therapy.

Causes

➤ The three main factors in the UK are:
  — diabetes mellitus
  — hypertension
  — ageing.

Classification[1]

Stage	eGFR	Description	Typical GFR testing frequency
1	>90	Normal or increased GFR, with other evidence of kidney damage	12 monthly
2	60–89	Slight decrease in GFR, with other evidence of kidney damage	12 monthly
3a	45–59	Moderate decrease in GFR, with or without other evidence of kidney damage	6 monthly
3b	30–44		6 monthly
4	15–29	Severe decrease in GFR, with or without other evidence of kidney damage	3 monthly
5	<15	Established renal failure	6 weekly

Assessment
➤ History and physical examination may identify the underlying diagnosis.
➤ First line investigations include:
  — urea and electrolytes
  — eGFR
  — random blood glucose
  — serum calcium and phosphate
  — full blood count
  — urinalysis for haematuria
  — urine ACR (albumin creatinine ratio).
➤ Further tests would depend on the results of these preliminary investigations (e.g. renal ultrasound, autoantibody screen, serum electrophoresis, urine for Bence Jones protein).

Management
➤ Prevention of development of chronic kidney disease in at risk patient groups is key.
➤ Aims of treatment in established cases:
  — identifying and treating underlying cause/s
  — reducing progression of kidney disease, e.g. addition of ACEIs or ARBs
  — addressing cardiovascular risk
  — relieving symptoms
  — managing complications, e.g. anaemia, bone disease.
➤ Consideration of dialysis in end-stage disease:
  — a decision to withhold dialysis should not be made on the basis of age alone.

National Institute for Health and Clinical Excellence: chronic kidney disease – key priorities for implementation[1]
1 To detect and identify proteinuria, preferentially by urine ACR.
2 Offer ACEIs/ARBs to non-diabetic people with CKD and hypertension and ACR >30 mg/mmol.
3 Nephrology referral should be considered for people with CKD in the following groups:
  — stage 4 and 5 CKD (with or without diabetes)

— higher levels of proteinuria (ACR >70 mg/mmol) unless known to be due to diabetes and already appropriately treated

— proteinuria (ACR >30 mg/mmol) with haematuria

— rapidly declining eGFR (>5 mL/min/1.73 m^2 in 1 year or >10 mL/min/1.73 m^2 within 5 years)

— poorly controlled hypertension despite use of at least four antihypertensive agents at therapeutic doses

— rare or genetic causes of CKD

— suspected renal artery stenosis.

4 Testing for CKD should be offered to people with the following risk factors:

— diabetes

— hypertension

— cardiovascular disease (ischaemic heart disease, chronic heart failure, peripheral vascular disease and cerebrovascular disease)

— structural renal tract disease, renal calculi or prostatic hypertrophy

— multisystem diseases with potential renal involvement

— family history of stage 5 CKD or hereditary kidney disease

— opportunistic detection of proteinuria or haematuria.

REFERENCE

1 National Institute for Health and Clinical Excellence. *Chronic Kidney Disease: early identification and management of chronic kidney disease in adults in primary and secondary care: NIHCE Clinical Guideline 73*. London: NIHCE; 2008. Available at: www.nice.org.uk/cg73 (accessed 25 May 2010).

FURTHER READING

Department of Health. *National Service Framework for Renal Services. Part One: dialysis and transplantation*. London: Department of Health; 2005. www.dh.gov.uk

Department of Health. *National Service Framework for Renal Service. Part Two: chronic kidney disease, acute renal failure and end of life care*. London: Department of Health; 2005. www.dh.gov.uk

CHAPTER 38

Thyroid disorders

HYPOTHYROIDISM
Prevalence
➤ Estimates vary depending on populations studied and criteria used – reported figures: 2.4–14%.

Causes
➤ Auto-immune thyroiditis.
➤ Post thyroidectomy.
➤ Following radioactive iodine treatment.
➤ Hypopituitarism (rare).

Symptoms and signs
➤ Vary – some individuals may present with non-specific atypical symptoms, while others present with classical features.
➤ Typical symptoms – dry skin, hair loss, lassitude, constipation, cold intolerance and weight increase despite anorexia. Untreated hypothyroidism may progress to confusion, psychoses and coma, which may be precipitated by hypothermia. Other symptoms include hypoguesia and dysguesia, impaired hearing and ataxia.
➤ Typical signs – coarsening of facial features, puffiness of face and eyes, loss of hair, particularly at the lateral aspect of eyebrows, puffiness of hands and feet, yellow skin due to carotinaemia, bradycardia, slow relaxing reflexes, effusions in serous cavities, i.e. pleura, pericardium.

Investigations
➤ Diagnosis confirmed by low thyroxine (T4) in the presence of raised thyroid stimulating hormone (TSH).
➤ Other abnormalities that may be noted include anaemia, which can be macrocytic or normochromic and normocytic, hyponatraemia, raised creatine kinase (CK) in patients with myopathy and mild abnormality of liver function tests (LFTs).

Management
➤ Levothyroxine – recommended starting dose 0.025 mg/day followed by increased dose every 4–6 weeks by 0.025 mg until euthyroid.
➤ Tri-iodothyronine recommended initially in a patient with coma or psychoses.
➤ In older patients on replacement therapy serum TSH level should be estimated once or twice a year.

Subclinical hypothyroidism
➤ 5% of population.
➤ Characterised by T4 at the lower end of normal with moderately raised TSH.
➤ Those with thyroid antibodies are more likely to progress to clinical hypothyroidism and therefore require follow up.
➤ Only some patients with subclinical hypothyroidism show improvement with therapy.

HYPERTHYROIDISM
Prevalence
➤ General population in the UK of around 2.7% in females (10-fold less in males) and of undiagnosed disease is around 0.5% in women.

Causes
➤ Multinodular goite.
➤ Plummer's disease.
➤ Graves' disease.
➤ Thyroiditis.
➤ Ectopic hormone production by tumour.

Clinical features
➤ No symptoms to classical symptoms and signs of thyrotoxicosis.
➤ Classical symptoms include tremor, nervousness, goitre, muscle weakness with cramps, weight loss, diarrhoea, abdominal pain, nausea, atrial fibrillation with or without heart failure, oedema of legs.
➤ Apathetic thyrotoxicosis – absence of sympathetic activation symptoms – present with lethargy, depression and weight loss.

Investigations
➤ Raised T4 and/or T3 with low TSH.
➤ Other abnormalities that may be noted include abnormal LFTs, mildly raised calcium.

Management
➤ Thionamides: carbimazole – starting dose 15–40 mg/day with maintenance dose of 5 mg/day once euthyroid.
➤ Radioactive iodine-131.
➤ Surgery reserved for large goitre that is producing pressure symptoms.
➤ Anticoagulation with warfarin should be considered in older subjects with thyrotoxicosis complicated by atrial fibrillation.
➤ B-adrenergic blockers, which act promptly to reduce symptoms and signs of tremor and to improve tachycardia and associated palpitation, may be useful in addition to thionamides in the management of thyrotoxicosis, particularly in cases of thyroiditis or mild cases of toxic nodular hyperthyroidism before radioiodine therapy.

Subclinical hyperthyroidism
➤ The prevalence of 'subclinical' hyperthyroidism (a biochemical diagnosis characterized by a low serum TSH with normal serum thyroid hormone concentrations) vary from 0.8–5.8%.
➤ There is only limited evidence to suggest that subclinical hyperthyroidism is associated with significant symptoms but there is a growing body of evidence that

low serum TSH is associated with adverse effects, particularly on heart and bone and this has led to a trend towards treatment of this condition.

Sick euthyroid syndrome

➤ Clinical euthyroid state with abnormal thyroid function tests.
➤ Ocurs with acute illness, paricularly in critically ill patient.
➤ Abnormalities of TFTs include low TSH with a decline in T4 and T3 levels.
➤ Associated with increasing mortality rates in critical care patients.
➤ Abnormalities return to normal after acute illness has resolved.

CHAPTER 39

Haematological disorders

ANAEMIA

Definition

➤ Anaemia is defined by the World Health Organization as a haemoglobin concentration of less than 13 g/dL in men and of less than 12 g/dL in women.[1]

Statistics

➤ The most common haematological abnormality in older people.
➤ Prevalence increases with age.
➤ Affects 20–25% of people aged over 65.
➤ Most common in men over 85 years.
➤ Not a normal consequence of ageing.

Associations

➤ Increased risk of mortality and morbidity.
➤ Falls.
➤ Heart failure.
➤ Delirium.
➤ Cognitive impairment.

Common types

Anaemia of chronic disease

➤ The most common form of anaemia in older people.
➤ Due to impaired ability to use iron in the reticuloendothelial system.
➤ Haemoglobin rarely drops below 10 g/dL.
➤ Disease associations include chronic infections and chronic inflammatory disorders.
➤ Usually normocytic although microcytosis may be present.
➤ Differentiated from iron deficiency by normal/high serum ferritin level.
➤ Treatment involves management of the underlying disorder.

Iron deficiency anaemia

➤ The second most common type of anaemia in older people.
➤ Usually secondary to gastrointestinal blood loss.
➤ Dietary deficiency of iron is uncommon.
➤ Characterised by a low serum ferritin level.
➤ Management involves identifying and treating the underlying cause, oral iron replacement and consideration of blood transfusion.

Megaloblastic anaemia
➤ Usually secondary to deficiencies of folic acid or vitamin B_{12}.
➤ Folic acid deficiency is generally due to insufficient oral intake.
➤ Vitamin B_{12} deficiency results largely from reduced intestinal absorption – pernicious anaemia is the most common cause in older people.
➤ Supplementation is the mainstay of therapy.

Other types of anaemia
➤ Anaemia associated with renal failure.
➤ Aplastic anaemia.
➤ Haemolytic anaemia.
➤ Bone marrow infiltration.
➤ Thalassaemia.
➤ Sickle cell trait.

CHRONIC LYMPHOCYTIC LEUKAEMIA
➤ Caused by a neoplastic proliferation of lymphocytes (B-cells in 95% of cases).
➤ Largely affects the older population.
➤ More common in men.
➤ Common presenting symptoms include lethargy secondary to anaemia and bruising due to thrombocytopaenia.
➤ Some patients may be asymptomatic.
➤ Lymphadenopathy and splenomegaly may be detected on clinical examination.
➤ Diagnosis is confirmed by lymphocytosis and lymphocytic infiltration of the bone marrow.
➤ Management includes supportive care as well as chemotherapy and radiation treatment in suitable cases.

MYELODYSPLASIA
➤ Characterised by varying degrees of anaemia, leucopaenia and thrombocytopaenia secondary to ineffective haematopoiesis.
➤ Most commonly occurs in people aged over the age of 70.
➤ May be an incidental finding.
➤ Symptomatic patients present with features suggestive of bone marrow failure – anaemia, bleeding, recurrent infection.
➤ Macrocytosis may be present.
➤ Diagnosis is made by bone marrow aspirate/biopsy.
➤ Some cases may be indolent whereas others have a poor prognosis with a high risk of progression to leukaemia.
➤ Asymptomatic patients do not require specific treatment but do need monitoring.
➤ Supportive treatments for those who are symptomatic include red cell and platelet transfusions.
➤ Other forms of therapy that may be appropriate in some circumstances include haematopoietic growth factors, immunosuppressants, immunomodulatory drugs and epigenetic agents.

MYELOMA
➤ A plasma cell malignancy.
➤ Peak incidence is 65–70 years.
➤ More common in men.
➤ Can result in anaemia, leucopaenia and thrombocytopaenia.

➤ Other complications include renal failure, hypercalcaemia and pathological fractures.

➤ A raised ESR, paraprotein on serum electrophoresis and urinary Bence Jones protein are typical findings.

➤ Diagnostic confirmation can be achieved via skeletal survey and bone marrow examination.

➤ Treatment includes supportive measures and in appropriate cases, chemotherapy, radiotherapy, immunosuppressants and biological therapies.

MONOCLONAL GAMMOPATHY OF UNDETERMINED SIGNIFICANCE

➤ A condition where abnormal plasma cells produce excess amounts of a monoclonal immunoglobulin.

➤ There is, however, no evidence of myeloma (renal failure, hypercalcaemia and pathological fractures are not features).

➤ Incidence increases with age.

➤ More common in men.

➤ Most cases are diagnosed incidentally as patients are asymptomatic.

➤ 1% per year risk of progression to malignancy and so annual follow-up is required.

REFERENCE

1 World Health Organization. Nutritional anaemias. Report of a WHO scientific group. *World Health Organ Tech Rep Ser.* 1968; **405**: 5–37.

CHAPTER 40

Common skin rashes and skin cancers

Rhodri Edwards

ECZEMA/DERMATITIS
➤ Inflammatory disorder of skin affecting the epidermis.
➤ Sub-acute eczema presents as an ill-defined itchy rash with erythematous, scaly patches, oedema and crusting. In acute eczema vesicles and bullae may be present. Scratching may cause excoriations.
➤ Chronic eczema is less exudative, scaly and lichenified.
➤ Atopic eczema has a strong genetic component and is associated with a history of asthma or hay fever.
➤ Commonly affects the flexure surfaces. In pigmented skin a reverse pattern of extensor involvement may be present.
➤ May be complicated by bacterial infection (*Staphylococcus aureus* and *Streptococcus pyogenes*) and most seriously herpes simplex (eczema herpeticum).

Management
➤ Avoid irritants/allergens.
➤ Emollients.
➤ Topical steroids.
➤ Antihistamines.
➤ Anti-infective agents.
➤ Immunosuppressive therapy.

Contact dermatitis/eczema
➤ Direct irritant contact dermatitis associated with external irritants such as soaps, detergents and solvents. Common in housewives, cleaners and hairdressers.
➤ Allergic contact dermatitis – a delayed type IV hypersensitivity reaction. Common examples include a nickel allergy to jewellery and latex allergy.
➤ Management involves stopping irritant or allergen, emollients and topical steroids.

Adult seborrhoeic eczema
➤ Erythematous, fine scaling rash affecting the scalp and face and less often the front and back of the chest, groin and axillae.

➤ Results from an overgrowth of *Pityrosporium ovale* and an immune response.
➤ Associated with Parkinson's disease and HIV.

Management
➤ Imidazole shampoos.
➤ A combination of mild steroid ointment and topical antifungal.

Discoid (nummular) eczema
➤ Well demarcated, coin-shaped, vesicular, weeping or scaly pink patches. Occur on limbs of middle-aged and the old. May be associated with stress.

Lichen simplex/nodular pruigo
➤ Lichen simplex: thickened flesh coloured/pink, hyperpigmented, scaly plaque resulting from continued rubbing and scratching. Associated with anxiety or stress.
➤ Nodular pruigo: itchy papules or domed nodules often found on upper trunk or extensor surfaces of limbs.
➤ Can be treated with potent topical steroids or intralesional steroid.

Varicose/gravitational eczema
➤ Chronic, patchy, eczematous rash of the lower legs associated with chronic venous hypertension. Brownish pigmentation (haemosiderin) may be seen. A history of venous thromboembolism, varicose veins or venous leg ulcers is common.
➤ Management involves emollients, elevation of legs, support stockings or compression bandaging, diuretics and topical steroids.

OTHER PAPULOSQUAMOUS DISORDERS
Psoriasis
➤ Chronic, hyperproliferative condition of epidermis affecting 1–2% of population.
➤ Late-onset psoriasis affects people aged 50–60.
➤ Well-demarcated erythematous/salmon-pink plaques with characteristic silvery-white scale.
➤ Commonly affects extensor surfaces of elbows, knees, buttocks and scalp.
➤ Nail involvement with pitting and onycholysis.
➤ Koebner's phenomenon.
➤ Other patterns include:
 — flexural psoriasis tends to occur in older people
 — guttate psoriasis – multiple small, round, red macules occur on trunk and become scaly. Precipitated by streptococcal tonsillitis
 — pustular psoriasis – localised (affecting palms or soles) or generalised
 — erythrodermic psoriasis.
➤ Associated with sero-negative arthritis (5%), HIV, alcohol abuse and may be precipitated by drugs (e.g. β-blockers, ACE inhibitors, lithium) and infections.

Management
➤ Emollients.
➤ Topical steroids.
➤ Vitamin D (calcipotriol).
➤ Coal tar preparations.
➤ Dithranol (can be challenging to use as staining of skin and clothing).
➤ Vitamin A.
➤ Ultraviolet radiation (narrow band UVB).

➤ Photochemotherapy PUVA.
➤ Systemic treatment: retinoids, methotrexate, cyclosporin.

Pityriasis rosea

➤ A single, oval, red, scaly *herald* patch develops into widespread smaller salmon-pink patches with delicate scaling on torso and body.
➤ Characteristically follows a 'Christmas tree' pattern along dermatomal lines on torso.
➤ Cause unknown.
➤ Spontaneously resolves.

Lichen planus

➤ Violaceous (purple), intensely itchy, flat-topped papules. White streaky pattern on the surface (Wickham's striae).
➤ White lacy lines are found in mouth.
➤ Koebner's phenomenon.
➤ Can be precipitated by drugs or occur as part of graft-versus-host disease (GVHD).
➤ Associated with diabetes mellitus, hepatitis C and primary billiary cirrhosis.
➤ Treat with super potent topical steroids.

Granuloma annulare

➤ Clusters of itchy, slightly erythematous papules often in the form of a ring.
➤ Often affect dorsum of hand, elbows, ankles and knees.
➤ Associated with diabetes mellitus.

Lichen sclerosis et atrophicus

➤ Commoner in females.
➤ Atrophic, white or ivory, itchy, shiny skin with well-defined edge-affecting vulva, glans penis, foreskin and perineal area. Architecture of perineum may be distorted.
➤ Treatment with super potent topical steroids.
➤ Risk of squamous cell carcinoma in long-standing lesions.

ROSACEA

➤ Chronic inflammatory disease characterised by facial flushing, facial erythema, telangiectasia and transient papules and pustules. Phymatous rosacea causes hyperplasia of sebaceous glands and connective tissue. Often disfiguring (rhinophyma).

INFECTIONS AND INFESTATIONS
Cellulitis

➤ Usually caused by *Streptococcus pyogenes*.
➤ Hot, painful, red, swollen skin associated with fever. May develop pustules or vesicles.
➤ Associated with diabetes mellitus, alcoholism.
➤ Treatment with systemic antibiotics.

Skin manifestations of tuberculosis

➤ Lupus vulgaris characterised by solitary irregular red-brown plaque usually found on face or limb. Described as having an 'apple jelly' appearance when pressed with a glass slide.

Lyme disease

➤ Caused by spirochaete *Borrelia burgdorferi* and transmitted by tick from an animal reservoir (e.g. deer).
➤ Erythema migrans: an annular erythema spreading outwards from a central papule caused by a tick bite.
➤ Complications: cranial polyneuropathy, painful radiculopathy, meningitis, myocarditis, polyarthalgia.
➤ Treat with oral tetracycline or penicillin.

Herpes zoster

➤ Caused by reactivation of dormant *Varicella zoster* virus.
➤ Prodrome of tingling or pain.
➤ Erythema which rapidly develops into a unilateral, dermatomal vesicular rash.
➤ Vesicles become purulent, burst and crust. Scarring may occur.
➤ Risk of secondary infection with *Staphylococci*.
➤ Ocular: involving nasociliary ganglion of ophthalmic branch of trigeminal nerve. Needs ophthalmology review.
➤ Ramsay Hunt syndrome (involvement of geniculate ganglion resulting in facial nerve palsy). Vesicles may only be found by examining ears.
➤ Postherpatic neuralgia.
➤ Contagious to contacts who have not had chicken pox.

Management

➤ Aciclovir 800 mg five times a day if given early.
➤ Valaciclovir/fanciclovir may also be used.
➤ Systemic steroids may be used to reduce inflammation in Ramsay Hunt syndrome.
➤ Postherpatic neuralgia may be treated with amitryptiline, carbemazepine or topical capsaicin.

FUNGAL INFECTIONS
Dermatophyte infections: 'ring worm'

➤ Tinea is a superficial fungus that colonises keratin. It is caused by three main genera *Trichophyton*, *Microsporidium* and *Epidermophyton*. Identified by microscopy and fungal cultures of skin, hair and nail.
➤ Tinea capitis: patchy alopecia with red inflamed skin.
➤ Tinea corporis: ring worm of the body. Spreading itchy red patch with scaling at edges and often central clearing.
➤ Tinea cruris: itchy erythematous plaque affecting groin.
➤ Tinea pedis: itching rash and scaling between toes (athletes foot).
➤ Tinea manuum: affecting the hands.
➤ Tinea unguium: causes white crumbling dystrophic nails.

Management

➤ Topical antifungals: clotrimazole, microconazole, terbinafine.
➤ Systemic therapy (for tinea capitis and tinea of nails): griseofulvin, itraconazole, terbinefine.

Candidiasis

➤ Caused by the yeast *Candida albicans*.
➤ Risk factors: obesity, moisture and maceration, diabetes, use of broad-spectrum antibiotics.

- ➤ Common presentations:
  - — oral candidiais: white adhesive plaques in mouth
  - — candidal interigo: moist glazed erythema in flexures (groin, under breasts, arm pits). Satellite lesions appear as small circular areas of erythema with pustules at the advancing edge
  - — genital candidiasis: candida vulvovaginitis is characterised by vaginal itching, soreness and a creamy discharge. Pustules coalese with redness and swelling. Candida balanitis causes cream-coloured pustules with swelling and erythema affecting the penis.

Management
- ➤ Identify and treat predisposing causes.
- ➤ For mouth infections: nystatin suspension, amphotericin lozenges or miconazole gel.
- ➤ Topical antifungal agents: clotrimazole, miconazole.
- ➤ Oral agents: fluconazole.

Scabies
- ➤ Caused by the mite *Sarcoptes scebiei*. Transferred by close bodily contact. Female mites burrow through stratum corneum and lay eggs. Characterised by burrows – tortuous tracts affecting palmer side of fingers, wrist, palms and soles. Small red papules often appear. Intense itching which may be worse at night.
- ➤ Norwegian scabies – widespread crusted eruption, huge numbers of mites found. Can cause epidemics and outbreaks. Commonly affects the immunocompromised.

Management
- ➤ Topical scabicide, e.g. malathion 0.5%: apply to all areas of skin below neck and wash off after 24 hours. Reapply to hands if washed. A second application 1 week from the first is recommended. Permethrin 5% is an alternative.
- ➤ Laundry of clothing and sheets.
- ➤ Contacts need treatment: all family members and sexual contacts should be treated simultaneously.

AUTOIMMUNE AND BLISTERING DISEASES
Pemphigus
- ➤ Affects people in middle age (peak onset 60–70 years). Commoner in Ashkenazi Jews and Asian people.
- ➤ Uncommon autoimmune disease characterised by intra-epidermal flaccid blisters and painful denuded erosions appearing on mouth, genitalia or body.
- ➤ Mucous membranes are often affected and may be the presenting feature.
- ➤ Mortality 15–25%.
- ➤ Biopsy of lesion for histopathology and direct immunofluorescence.
- ➤ Serology for circulating antibodies.

Management
- ➤ High dose oral steroids.
- ➤ Immunosuppressive agents: azathioprine, cyclophosphamide, mycophenolate mofetil, cyclosporine.

Bullous pemphigoid
- ➤ Autoimmune disease affecting the dermo-epidermal junction characterised by large tense fluid filled blisters with an erythematous base.

➤ Starts on limbs and spreads to trunk.
➤ One-third of patients have oral lesions. Itchy.
➤ Vesicles rapidly enlarge and burst leaving eroded skin, sometimes with haemorrhagic scabs.
➤ Possible underlying malignancy.
➤ Biopsy for histopathology and immunofluorescence.
➤ Serology for circulating antibodies.

Management
➤ Oral steroids.
➤ Azathioprine used as a steroid-sparing agent.

Dermatitis herpetiformis
➤ Characterised by sub-epidermal excoriated vesicles and papules on the elbows, knees and buttocks.
➤ Intensely itchy.
➤ Deposits of IgA and C3 in dermal papillae along the basement membrane.
➤ Associated with coeliac disease (often subclinical) and rarely lymphoma of the bowel.

Management
➤ Dapsone.
➤ Gluten-free diet.

VASCULAR AND LYMPHATIC SKIN DISEASE
Raynaud's
➤ Paroxysmal condition of fingers and toes induced by cold.
➤ Presents as pallor and coolness followed by cyanosis and reactive hyperaemia.

Erythema ab igne
➤ Pigmented reticular erythema sometimes with blistering affecting the lower legs. Caused by thermal injury such as sitting too close to a fire.

Livedo reticularis
➤ Net-like pattern of dusky erythema occurring on limbs.
➤ Causes: idiopathic, polyarteritis nodosa, connective tissue disease, cryoglobulinaemia, thrombocythaemia, pancreatitis, TB, bacterial endocarditis, vascular disease.

Lymphoedema
➤ Chronic non-pitting oedema with secondary brawny changes affecting the lower limbs due to lymphatic insufficiency.
➤ Causes:
— primary underdevelopment of lymphatic system (e.g. Milroy's disease).
— secondary causes: surgical removal of lymph nodes, post radiotherapy, malignant disease, filarial infection, venous disease.

SKIN MANIFESTATIONS OF SYSTEMIC DISEASE
Pruritis/itching
➤ Unpleasant sensation that leads to desire to scratch the skin.
➤ May be associated with inflammatory skin disease (eczema, scabies, lichen planus, urticaeria, bullous disease) or a sign of systemic disease.

➤ Large number of conditions associated with itching; xerosis (dry skin), thyroid disease, iron deficiency, diabetes mellitus, haematological and solid organ malignancy, chronic renal disease, hepatobiliary disease, drugs (opiates, codeine and drugs causing cholestasis), psychiatric problems.

Management
➤ Topical treatments: emollients and soap substitutes, topical crotamiton, cooling preparations such as 1–3% menthol in aqueous cream.
➤ Antihistamines.
➤ Antidepressants.
➤ Others: topical capsaicin, gabapentin, opiate antagonists, thalidomide, phototherapy.

Erythema multiforme
➤ Annular non-scaling erythematous plaque with central clearing occurring symmetrically on palms, soles, forearms and legs. Often described as 'target' lesions.
➤ Causes:
  — viral infections (commonly herpes simplex but also EBV, orf, hepatitis A and B)
  — mycoplasma infection
  — others: drugs, connective tissue disease, malignancy.
➤ Stevens Johnson syndrome is a variant and is associated with fever, mucosal lesions and other organ involvement.
➤ Supportive treatment. Severe forms require hospitalisation and potentially ITU admission. Use of steroids is controversial.

Erythema nodosum
➤ Tender, dusky blue-red nodule commonly found on legs. May be associated with athralgia, malaise, fever.
➤ Causes: infection (bacteria: streptococcus, mycoplasma, TB, chlamydia), drugs, systemic disease (sarcoidosis, ulcerative colitis, Crohn's disease).
➤ Histologically: paniculitis.
➤ Lesions usually resolve in 6–8 weeks.

Pyoderma gangrenosum
➤ Erythematous nodules which ulcerate. Characteristic blue/black undermined edge and purulent surface.
➤ Associated with inflammatory bowel disease, rheumatoid arthritis, myeloma and lymphoproliferative disorders.

Acanthosis nigrans
➤ Thickened velvety hyperpigmented skin.
➤ Commonly found in axillae, neck and groin.
➤ Associated with obesity, insulin resistance and underlying malignancy.

Necrobiosis lipodica
➤ Well-defined erythematous plaque, which becomes yellow, waxy and atrophic. Occurs on shins.
➤ Associated with diabetes mellitus.

Sarcoidosis
➤ Lupus pernio – violaceous plaque affecting nose or ears.
➤ Red-brown papules and plaques may be present on trunk and limbs.
➤ Erythema nodosum seen in acute sarcoidosis.

Thyroid disease
➤ Pre-tibial myxoedema: a red-brown waxy plaque on shin. Associated with Grave's disease.

CONNECTIVE TISSUE DISEASE
Lupus erythematosus
➤ Chronic discoid lupus erythematosus presents as well-defined erythematous, scaly plaques with telangiectasia and follicular plugging affecting sun-exposed areas (commonly the face). Causes scarring alopecia.
➤ Only 5% have systemic lupus erythematosus.
➤ Treatment with high-factor sunscreens, topical steroids and antimalarials. Oral steroids and immunosuppressive agents may be used.
➤ Systemic lupus erythematosus: butterfly rash, macular popular eruption, palmer erythema, vasculitis, Raynaud's phenomenon, livedo reticularis and purura.

Scleroderma
➤ Dermatological changes occur in limited cutaneous scleroderma and diffuse cutaneous scleroderma. They include Raynaud's phenomenon, digital ulcers, telangiectasia, digital ischaemia, tight skin over fingers and face causing beak-like nose and microstomia.
➤ Morphea (localised to skin) presents with purple, mauve indurated skin. Mature lesions have waxy centre with lilac-coloured edge.

Dermatomyositis
➤ 'Heliotrope rash': magenta-coloured rash around eyes.
➤ Gottron's papules: purple papules over knuckles.
➤ Ragged cuticles.
➤ Part of an immunological disorder with profound proximal muscle weakness, Raynaud's phenomenon and other systemic features.
➤ Associated with underlying malignancy in 15–25% of cases.
➤ Treatment with systemic steroids and immunosuppressive agents.

DRUG ERUPTIONS
➤ 2% of hospital patients develop a drug rash.
➤ More common in women and with increasing age.

TABLE 40.1 Drug eruption and commonly associated drugs

Drug eruption	Drugs commonly associated
Mobilliform rash	ACE inhibitors, allopurinol, amoxicillin, anticonvulsants, thiazides, trimethoprim
Urticaeria and angioedem	ACE inhibitors (can occur after years), alendronate, aspirin, clopidogrel, penicillin, opiates, PPI
Lichenoid eruptions	Amlodipine, β-blockers, diltiazem, enalapril, frusemide, glimepiride, pravastatin, PPI, thiazides

(*continued*)

TABLE 40.1 (*cont.*)

Drug eruption	Drugs commonly associated
Eczematous eruptions	Allopurinol, anticonvulsants, aspirin, diltiazem, lithium, omeprazole
Photosensitive	ACE inhibitors, amioderone, diltiazem, frusemide, quinolones, sulphonamides, tetracyclines, thiazide
Small-vessel leucocytoclastic vasculitis	Aspirin/NSAIDs, allopurinol, penicillin, sulphonamide
Erythema multiforme/Stevens Johnson syndrome	Alfuzocin, allopurinol, anticonvulsants, isoniazid, lamotrigine, penicillins, phenytoin

SKIN CANCERS
Actinic keratoses
➤ Pre-malignant, discrete, rough-surfaced macules or papules occurring on chronically sun-exposed skin.
➤ Common on face, backs of hands and legs.
➤ Small risk of transmission to squamous cell carcinoma.

Management
➤ Photo-protective advice – appropriate clothing and sun hats, high factor sunscreen.
➤ Cryotherapy (freezing with liquid nitrogen), curettage and cautery, topical 5-fluorouracil.

Bowen's disease
➤ Intraepidermal carcinoma (no dermal invasion) occurring as slowly enlarging erythematous roughened patch.
➤ More common in women.
➤ May progress to squamous cell carcinoma (~3–5%).

Management
➤ Surgical excision or curettage, cryotherapy or topical 5-fluorouracil.

Squamous cell carcinoma
➤ Malignant tumour presenting as an indurated, crusted or scaling, nodule, papule or plaque that may ulcerate. Occurs on sun-damaged skin or mucous membranes.
➤ Marjolin's ulcer: ulcerating squamous cell carcinoma arising from areas of chronically inflamed or scarred skin such as ulcers.
➤ Causes include irradiation (sunlight most common), immunosuppressive therapy, human papilloma virus, chronic scarring conditions, carcinogens (polycyclic hydrocarbons).
➤ Locally invasive and risk of metastasis to lymph nodes and other organs.

Management
➤ Surgical excision.
➤ Radiotherapy.

Basal cell carcinoma
➤ Most common cancer in Europe, Australia and USA.
➤ Nodulocystic basal cell carcinoma is the most common type. Translucent,

pearl-coloured, dome-shaped papule that slowly enlarges with characteristic rolled, pearly edge. Often has surface telangiectasia and central ulceration.
➤ Morphoeic (slowly expanding, ill-defined, pearly, waxy plaques), superficial (slowly expanding, pink, scaly plaque commonly found on trunk) and pigmented types exist.
➤ Commonly found on sun-exposed areas of head or neck.
➤ Locally invasive but rarely metastasises.

Management
➤ Surgical excision.
➤ Mohs micrographic surgical technique – lesion is removed in stages with histological examination of surgical margins to ensure adequate excision.
➤ Radiotherapy.
➤ Photodynamic therapy.
➤ Imiquimod, topical 5-fluorouracil.

Malignant melanoma
➤ Incidence increasing.
➤ Risk factors: exposure to ultraviolet radiation, burning exposure during childhood, multiple pigmented naevi, fair 'celtic' skin type (red hair and freckles), family history of melanoma, sunbed use.
➤ 50% occur in pre-existing moles.
➤ Pigmented lesion which may have recently changed. Suspicious features include change in size or shape, increased growth, asymmetry, border irregularity, change in colour (deepening pigmentation), an inflamed red edge, bleeding, oozing or crusting and itching or pain.
➤ Four main types:
  — superficial spreading melanoma: flat, asymmetrical, varied pigmentation, irregular border
  — Hutchinson lentigo or lentigo maligna (melanoma): slow-growing, irregular pigmented patch commonly on sun-exposed face of older people. Progresses to melanoma
  — acral lentiginous melanoma: occurs on palms, soles and under nails
  — nodular melanoma.
➤ Special variants:
  — subungual melanoma
  — amelanotic melanoma: does not contain melanin.
➤ Risk of metastasis.

Management
➤ Surgical excision.
➤ Breslow's thickness and Clark's levels guide prognosis.
➤ Limited effective treatment for metastatic disease.

Mycosis fungoides
➤ Asymmetrical, variously shaped, scaly pink or red plaques and patches distributed over limbs and trunk.
➤ Cutaneous T-cell lymphoma.
➤ Treatment: PUVA, topical nitrogen mustard, local radiotherapy, chemotherapy regimens.

PART IV

Administrative aspects of services

CHAPTER 41

Health and social services

PRINCIPLES OF GOOD MEDICAL AND SOCIAL CARE FOR ELDERS (BRITISH GERIATRICS SOCIETY 2003)[1]
➤ Involvement of the older person in decisions on their future care.
➤ Promotion of good health.
➤ Prevention of illness.
➤ Reduction of disability.
➤ Provision of home support.
➤ Preservation of dignity, autonomy and respect.
➤ Elimination of age discrimination.

ACUTE MEDICAL CARE
Models of geriatric medicine
➤ Traditional – older adults with complex needs are admitted to the geriatric service.
➤ Age-defined – medical patients above a certain age are admitted under a geriatrician.
➤ Integrated – both older patients and younger adults are cared for by a general physician with an interest in geriatrics.
➤ No firm evidence is available to indicate which pattern of care provides the best outcome.

Aims
➤ Waiting time in the emergency department should be less than 4 hours before transfer or discharge.
➤ Inter-ward transfers should be minimal.
➤ Older patients admitted under a general medical team should see a geriatrician within 72 hours.
➤ Care should be delivered by an experienced multidisciplinary team skilled in dealing with the problems of old age.
➤ The need for rehabilitation should be identified as soon as possible.
➤ Discharge planning should commence early.
➤ Specialist opinions, investigations and treatment should not be compromised purely on the basis of age.

Specialist inpatient geriatric services
➤ Stroke – a specialist stroke service should be established in each trust.
➤ Orthogeriatrics – a pre- and postoperative care liaison service to include assessment of falls risk and bone protection should be available.

➤ General rehabilitation – either at the acute hospital site or other non-acute care facility.

INTERMEDIATE CARE

➤ A term that has been used in many different contexts.
➤ Born out of the National Beds Inquiry (2000), which emphasised the inappropriate use of many acute hospital beds.[2]
➤ Aims to promote recovery and independence following acute inpatient care provision or as an alternative to acute medical admission.
➤ Encompasses a range of services including:
  — rapid response
  — supported discharge
  — inpatient rehabilitation
  — hospital at home
  — day rehabilitation.
➤ Is the focus of Standard 3 of the National Service Framework for Older People.[3]

REHABILITATION

➤ A process aimed at enabling people to reach and maintain their optimal physical, sensory, intellectual, psychological and social functional levels, as well as providing the tools they need to attain independence and self-determination (World Health Organization).[4]
➤ Recovery from illness often takes longer in older people.
➤ Rehabilitation is an essential component of geriatric practice.
➤ Success relies on a multidisciplinary approach with effective communication between members of the team.
➤ Focus can be general or specific, e.g. stroke or orthogeriatric rehabilitation.
➤ Care can be provided in the inpatient setting or may be community based.
➤ Stages of the rehabilitation process (British Geriatrics Society 1997):[5]
  — Assessment – identification of problems
  — Planning – analysis of problems and goal setting
  — Treatment – intervention to reduce disability and handicap
  — Evaluation – assessment of effectiveness of intervention
  — Care – alleviation of any consequences of disability
  — Advice – development of coping strategies for patients and carers.

CONTINUING CARE

➤ NHS-funded hospital-based care for patients who have particularly difficult continuing medical, physical, psychological and emotional needs and in whom there is no potential for improvement.
➤ Rapid expansion in private care capacity over the last three decades means that nursing home places now outnumber continuing care beds by 2:1.
➤ National eligibility criteria for entry to continuing care facilities must be met.

RESPITE CARE

➤ Can be provided in the NHS or social service facilities depending on the patient's requirements.
➤ May be an isolated episode or part of a programme to relieve carer stress.
➤ A good opportunity to reassess the needs of both patients and carers.

OUTPATIENT CLINICAL CARE
➤ A means of seeking a non-urgent geriatric medical assessment.
➤ Clinics may be general or specialized, e.g. falls, memory, continence.
➤ Access to multidisciplinary advice/input should be available.
➤ Smooth running depends on reliable transport services for disabled patients.
➤ Long waiting times should be avoided.

GERIATRIC DAY HOSPITALS
➤ Originally developed in the UK in the 1960s.
➤ Benefits have been controversial for many years.
➤ May avoid admission to hospital or institutional care.
➤ Act as an interface between hospital and community services.
➤ Services provided include functional assessment, medical review and treatment if required and rehabilitation if appropriate.
➤ Patients attend for half/full days depending on need.
➤ Roles may extend to information provision, health education, respite for carers and opportunity for social interaction.

NHS COMMUNITY SERVICES
Services include:
➤ District nursing.
➤ Physiotherapy.
➤ Occupational therapy.
➤ Continence advice.
➤ Speech and language therapy.
➤ Dietetics.
➤ Podiatry.

DOMICILIARY VISITS
➤ A visit to a patient's home by a specialist, normally a consultant, at the request of the GP and normally in his or her company, to advise on the diagnosis or treatment of a patient who, on medical grounds, cannot attend the hospital.
➤ In reality, joint visits rarely occur.
➤ Advantages:
  — may avoid inappropriate admissions
  — provide valuable information about the home circumstances.
➤ Criticisms:
  — time consuming
  — abuse of the system through inappropriate referrals.

PSYCHOGERIATRIC SERVICES
➤ Specialist mental health services for older people have expanded over recent years.
➤ Services include:
  — psychogeriatric inpatient care
  — old age psychiatry and care of the old inpatient liaison
  — outpatient clinics including specialised services, e.g. memory
  — long-stay institutional care (NHS and private facilities)
  — community-based assessment and treatment
  — domiciliary visits
  — outreach visits to nursing and residential homes.

SOCIAL SERVICES

➤ Social care encompasses a wide range of services provided by local authorities and the private sector including home care assistance, meals on wheels, day centres and residential/nursing home facilities.

➤ The Care Standards Act (2000)[6] was developed as part of the government's plan to modernise social care by regulating all social care services including care homes in accordance with national minimum standards.

LONG-TERM PLACEMENT

➤ If a patient is unable to return home after treatment and rehabilitation, they may expect to receive care in another setting depending on their needs.

➤ Alternative types of accommodation include sheltered housing, residential care, nursing home care or long-stay wards in hospital.

CARE HOMES

➤ Old people in care homes can be very vulnerable.

➤ The Royal College of Physicians has established a set of guidelines designed to optimise their care:[7]
  — a standardised interdisciplinary approach to assessment, care planning and care delivery should be adopted
  — all practitioners engaged in care home services should have appropriate training
  — a geriatrics nurse specialist and GP with a special interest in care of the old should play key roles
  — consultant outreach sessions would be useful.

REFERENCES

1 British Geriatrics Society. *Standards of Medical Care for Older People: Expectations and Recommendations. Compendium Document A3* (revised January 2003). London: British Geriatrics Society; 1997. Available at: www.bgs.org.uk/Publications/Compendium/compend_1-3.htm (accessed 25 May 2010).

2 Department of Health. *National Beds Inquiry*. London: Department of Health; 2000. Available at: http://webarchive.nationalarchives.gov.uk/+/www.dh.gov.uk/en/Publications andstatistics/Publications/AnnualReports/Browsable/DH_4989760 (accessed 25 May 2010).

3 Department of Health. *National Service Framework for Older People*. London: Department of Health; 2001. Available at: www.dh.gov.uk (accessed 25 May 2010).

4 World Health Organization. *Rehabilitation*. Geneva: World Health Organization; 2010. Available at: www.who.int/topics/rehabilitation/en (accessed 25 May 2010).

5 British Geriatrics Society. *Rehabilitation of Older People. Compendium document A4*. London: British Geriatrics Society; 1997. Available at: www.bgs.org.uk/Publications/Compendium/compend_1-4.htm (accessed 25 May 2010).

6 Department of Health. *Explanatory Notes to Care Standards Act*. London: Department of Health; 2000. Available at: www.opsi.gov.uk/acts/acts2000/en/ukpgaen_20000014_en_1.htm (accessed 25 May 2010).

7 Royal College of Physicians. *The Health and Care of Older People in Care Homes. Working Party Report*. London: RCP; 2000. www.rcplondon.ac.uk

CHAPTER 42

Orthogeriatric services

➤ Trauma is the fifth most common cause of mortality in people aged over 65.
➤ Hip fracture is the major cause of this mortality and also causes significant morbidity.
➤ 80% of hip fractures occur in females above 65 years of age.

These patients frequently present with complex age related physiological processes together with the effects of chronic illnesses. The majority require surgery, which predisposes them to a range of postoperative complications.

Several models of collaborative care exist between orthopaedic and geriatric specialities for the management of older trauma patients. These collaborative schemes have led to the development of orthogeriatric services. A number of different models exist. Most models involve a geriatrician and the multidisciplinary team and have been shown to be beneficial for older patients who require rehabilitation following hip surgery.

ROLE OF THE ORTHOGERIATRIC SERVICE

The aim of an orthogeriatric service is to optimise medical management so that complications are prevented, appropriate treatments given, functional outcomes improved, discharge is facilitated and mortality and morbidity are reduced.

MODELS OF ORTHOGERIATRIC CARE

➤ *Traditional orthopaedic care*: the older patient with a fracture is admitted to a trauma ward and their care and rehabilitation is managed by the orthopaedic team. Geriatrician input varies from a consultative service for referrals, regular geriatrician ward rounds or multidisciplinary ward rounds with medical and surgical teams.
➤ *Geriatric Orthopaedic Rehabilitation Unit* (GORU): perioperative care is under the orthopaedic team and the patient is transferred early postoperatively to a geriatric rehabilitation unit. Selection of patients for transfer may be by the orthopaedic team, a specialist liaison nurse or geriatrician. The extent of orthopaedic input after transfer is variable but should be at least weekly. There is some evidence that this model increases length of stay and may not be cost-effective.
➤ *Orthogeriatric liaison nurse/hip fracture nurse*: this is usually a senior nurse who takes responsibility for the patient throughout the course of their clinical care, coordinating initial assessment, facilitating preoperative work-up, supervising postoperative care, rehabilitation, discharge planning, secondary prevention and follow-up.
➤ *Combined orthogeriatric care*: the fracture patient is admitted to a specialised orthogeriatric ward under joint care of the geriatrician and orthopaedic surgeon. This degree of collaboration is essential for an integrated Hip Fracture Service

with early preoperative assessment by the geriatric team who will also lead the multidisciplinary postoperative care. Rehabilitation may take place in this setting or in a separate unit depending on local availability.

➤ *Early supported discharge and community rehabilitation*: intermediate care rehabilitation schemes have been developed in a number of areas that allow patients to be discharged earlier from the acute setting either for ongoing rehabilitation in their own homes or in a dedicated facility in the community.

The benefits of an orthogeriatric liasion service include:
➤ Improved medical care in the pre- and perioperative period.
➤ Optimising patient care preoperatively reducing delays to surgery.
➤ Earlier recognition and intervention when complications occur reducing morbidity and mortality.
➤ Better communication with patients, relatives and carers.
➤ Improved communication and working of the multidisciplinary team.
➤ Reduction in adverse events.
➤ Earlier and more appropriate initiation of rehabilitation.
➤ Assessment and secondary prevention of falls and fractures.
➤ Improved discharge planning and use of discharge resources.
➤ Reduced length of stay.
➤ Education and training of surgical, medical and professions allied to medicine teams.
➤ Audit.

There is still no definite consensus on the preferred or best model and to date it has largely been developed according to local need and expertise. There is increasing National Guidance and recommendations. The National Service Framework for Older People recommends that at least one general ward in an acute hospital should be developed as a centre of excellence for orthogeriatric practice, and that the particular type of orthogeriatric collaboration should be agreed at a local level. The revised edition of the Blue Book, sponsored by the British Orthopaedic Association and the British Geriatrics Society summarises current best practice in the care and secondary prevention of fragility fractures and recommends early involvement of the geriatrician and multidisciplinary team. The proposed best practice tariff for fractured neck of femur, due in April 2010, is likely to specify joint care with involvement of a geriatrician from admission.

FURTHER READING

Cameron I *et al*. Geriatric rehabilitation following fractures in older people: a systematic review. *Health Technol Assess*. 2000; **4**(2).

Scottish Intercollegiate Guidelines Network. *Management of Hip Fracture in Older People. SIGN guidelines 111*. Edinburgh: SIGN; 2009.

British Orthopaedic Association. *The Care of Patients with Fragility Fracture* (The Blue Book). London: British Orthopaedic Association; 2007. www.fractures.com/pdf/BOA-BGS-Blue-Book.pdf

National Hip Fracture Database (NHFD). www.nhfd.co.uk

CHAPTER 43

Income maintenance

PENSIONS
State Pension

➤ The amount of basic State Pension one receives depends upon the qualifying years one has built up before reaching State Pension age (60 for females and 65 for males. This will be equalized to 65 between 2010 and 2020 – women born on or before 5 April 1950 will not be affected by the change, but those born between 6 April 1950 and 5 April 1955 will be allowed to have a State Pension between the age of 60 and 65).

➤ A man will receive the full State Pension if he has 44 years of qualifying years.

➤ From April 2010 the full basic pension will be £97.65 a week for a single person and £156.15 for a couple.

➤ For a female, 39 qualifying years are required in order to get the full basic pension – this rule applies until 2010, when 30 years of qualifying years will be needed to qualify for a full pension.

➤ People who do not qualify for the full basic State Pension but who have more than 25% of qualifying years will get an approximate pro rata weekly income based on number of qualifying years. For those reaching retirement age on or after 6 April 2010 for each qualifying year an individual will get a thirtieth of the full amount for each qualifying year.

➤ For those aged 80 years who do not have a State Pension, there is a non-contributory State Pension provided the person lives in the UK, has lived in the UK for a total of 10 years or more in any continuous period of 20 years after their 60th birthday and has no basic State Pension, or less than 60% of the full rate.

➤ Individual can defer claiming State Pension – deferral for at least 5 weeks will increase the State Pension by 1%.

State Second Pension

➤ This replaced State Earnings-Related Pension Scheme (SERPS) in April 2002.

➤ SERPS was based on amount of National Insurance contributions and amount of money earned.

➤ The State Second Pension provides generous additional state pension to low or moderate earners, people with long-term illness or disability and carer of disabled people who spend at least 20 hours a week.

➤ Individuals can opt out of the additional state pension if he/she is in a private pension scheme.

Occupational pensions
➤ Most employers offer some kind of pension scheme and if an employer does not offer a company scheme and employs over five employees they must offer access to a stakeholder pension.
➤ Most schemes have retirement age of 60 or 65, but allow individual to collect pension from age of 50. From 2010 this figure will be raised to 55.
➤ An individual can collect pension and continue to work for the same employer.

Pension credit
Pension credit guarantees that everyone aged 60 and over has an income of at least:
➤ £132.60 per week for a single person aged 60 or over but under 65, and this rises to £181.00 for those over 65.
➤ £202.40 or couples if one is aged 60 and both are under 65 and £266.00 if both are over 65.

Higher entitlement for those who are severely disabled and live alone or with another severely disabled person, those who are carers and are entitled to Carer's Allowance or Housing Benefit.

Pension credit consists of two elements – a guarantee credit element highlighted above and a savings credit element. The latter is paid if a single person has a total income from pensions, savings, investments and earnings of between £96 and £181 a week and a couple's joint income is between £153.40 and £266.00. The maximum savings credit paid is £20.40 per week for a single person and £27.03 for a couple.

Annuities
➤ An annuity by definition is an exchange of a pension lump sum in return for an income from an insurance company.
➤ Once the annuity has been purchased a person cannot ever get the lump sum back.
➤ An annuity can be purchased any time between the ages of 50 and 75. The annuity rates depend upon the person's life expectancy, the amount in the pension fund and the economic conditions at the time of purchase.
➤ Compulsory purchase annuities relate to pension funds and the rules state that a person must purchase an annuity with his/her pension fund (net of any tax-free cash entitlement) by a maximum age of 75.
➤ Pensioners who do not buy annuity but choose to draw income from the pension fund after the age of 75 will now have the fund taxed by up to 70% when they die.
➤ Purchased life annuities relate to non-pension monies and allow someone with a lump sum of capital to convert that to a regular income for life if they wish.
➤ Basic conventional annuities have a number of different options (see below).

Level annuities – fixed level annuities
➤ These pay a guaranteed fixed level of income for life.
➤ Disadvantage of a level annuity – it provides no insurance against inflation and it allows the annuitant's income to fall steadily further behind average incomes if there is economic growth. For this reason potential annuitants might be better advised to purchase index-linked or escalating annuities.

Escalating annuities
➤ Payment increases every year, although initially the income will start at a lower level and will take a number of years before it reaches the amount available from a level annuity.

Spouse's pension

➤ This option allows someone to ensure that their spouse will continue to enjoy an income (typically 50%) after their death. Again this will usually mean a lower starting pension because of the probability that the annuity provider will be paying out for longer.

Guaranteed period

➤ This allows a person to have their pension paid for a guaranteed minimum period even if they die during this period. Typically the options are either 5 or 10 years.
➤ There are also other types of annuities.

Section 32 annuities

➤ Also known as Section 32 buyouts.
➤ Allow people to transfer company pension scheme benefits to a private fund.

Income drawdown

➤ Allows a person to draw any tax-free cash entitlement and then draw an income between government set guidelines, which can be varied depending on your requirements.

Impaired annuities/enhanced annuities

➤ Allow higher annuity rates if an individual is suffering or has suffered from a number of medical conditions that could shorten life expectancy, e.g. high blood pressure, cancer, strokes, heart attacks, Parkinson's disease, Alzheimer's disease, etc.

Immediate annuities

➤ Enable a person to draw income from their pension fund now rather than at a future date.

Purchase life annuities

➤ These allow one to purchase an annuity from funds that did not originate from a pension fund, i.e. non-pension savings. They work in much the same way as an annuity from a pension but with one notable and extremely beneficial difference.
➤ Under pension rules the annuity a person receives from a pension fund is treated as taxable income in the same way as income from normal employment would be. However, if a person uses other monies to buy a purchased life annuity, the tax treatment is different – some of the income received is treated as capital, which is not taxed, and therefore the tax burden is reduced.
➤ The other benefit of purchase life annuity is that it reduces the value of estate and thus size of estate for inheritance.

Care fee annuities

➤ These new annuities aim to provide a guaranteed income in return for a lump sum to pay for care in a residential or nursing home.

OTHER BENEFITS/ALLOWANCES AVAILABLE FOR OLDER PEOPLE
Winter Fuel Payment

➤ £250.00 for those aged 60 and over.
➤ £400.00 for those aged 80 or over.

Warm Front Scheme in England
➤ Warm Front grant for paying for heating and insulation improvements in privately owned or rented home.
➤ Anyone 60 or over who is receiving pension credit, housing benefit or council tax benefit may be eligible.
➤ £3 500 or up to £6 000 if home needs oil central heating.

Housing Benefit (rent allowance/rent rebate)
➤ This helps towards rent.
➤ It is paid by local councils – the maximum available is the eligible rent.
➤ To obtain this a person does not need to get any other benefit.
➤ It does not cover mortgage interest.

Claiming in advance
➤ Housing benefit is determined by:
  — savings a person and their partner have
  — money that is coming in the form of earnings, some benefits, occupational pension and tax credit.

The other factors that will be taken into account by the local council are:
➤ the amount of rent for the particular
➤ the home is a reasonable size for the person and their partner
➤ the area the home is in.

The decision made by the council can be challenged and appeal made to an independent appeal tribunal administered by the Appeal Service Agency.

Attendance Allowance (AA)
➤ This benefit is paid if a person becomes ill or disabled on or after their 65th birthday.
➤ The rate of payment is dependent upon the care needs during the day, during the night or both.
➤ The AA can be claimed even if no one is actually giving the care.
➤ It is not affected by savings or other money an older person is getting.
➤ No medical examination is necessary.
➤ The amount paid is:
  — higher rate £71.40 per week
  — lower rate £47.80 per week.
➤ Payment of AA usually stops 4 weeks after an individual goes into a residential care or nursing home and this is arranged by social services. If the move is arranged by an individual and they are paying for the care, then they can continue to receive the AA.
➤ If a person has a progressive disease and is not expected to live for more than another 6 months there are special rules for claiming to make sure benefit is received more quickly and easily.

Disability Living Allowance
➤ Paid to people who need help looking after themselves and people who find it difficult to walk and get around.
➤ It comprises two elements:
  — the care component:
    • lower rate £18.95 per week

- middle rate £47.80
- higher rate £71.40
— the mobility component:
  - lower rate £18.95 per week
  - higher rate £49.85 per week.
➤ Like Attendance Allowance it is not means tested. In April 2010, the figures will rise by 1.5%.

Carer's Allowance (CA)
➤ Paid to full-time carers aged 16 and over who are spending at least 35 hours a week looking after someone who is getting:
  — Attendance Allowance
  — Disability Living Allowance at the middle or highest rate for personal care
  — Industrial Injuries Disablement Benefit Constant Attendance Allowance
  — War Pensions Constant Attendance Allowance
➤ However, the carer cannot get the CA if they are in full-time education or earning above a certain amount.
➤ Carer's Allowance is taxable.
➤ Carer does not have to be related to, or live with, the person he/she is caring for.
➤ Carer's allowance from April 2010 will be £53.90.

Council Tax Benefit
➤ Can be claimed by a person aged 60 and over who has savings of less than £16 000 and is receiving guarantee credit of pension credit.

Community Care Grants
➤ Financial help to live independently in the community for those who are receiving pension credit and are considering moving out of residential and institutional care or need help to stay in his/her home and not go into a residential home.

Local bus passes
➤ Pass entitles an individual over 60 to free off-peak local bus travel anywhere in England.
➤ In Wales, individuals can travel anytime.
➤ Free local bus and long-distance coach within Scotland at any time of the day.

OTHER BENEFITS AVAILABLE
Free passports
➤ Eligible: those over 79 years of age if applied for a passport since 19 May 2004.

Free prescriptions and sight test
➤ Aged 60 and over.

Free TV licence
➤ Aged 75 and over.

FURTHER INFORMATION
Department for Work and Pensions www.dwp.gov.uk/directgov
Understanding the Basic State Pension www.direct.gov.uk/en/Pensionsandretirementplanning/
StatePension/Basicstatepension/DG_10014671

Benefits and Financial Support www.direct.gov.uk/en/MoneyTaxAndBenefits/Benefits
   TaxCreditsAndOtherSupport/index.htm
The Warm Front Scheme: a government funded initiative www.warmfront.co.uk/

CHAPTER 44

Audit, clinical governance and appraisal

➤ Audit is defined as the systematic critical analysis of the quality of clinical care, including procedures used for diagnosis and treatment, the use of resources, the resulting outcome and quality of life for the patient. The purpose of audit should be educational and relevant to patient care.

➤ To perform a successful audit cycle a systematic approach is essential, involving the stages outlined in Figure 44.1.

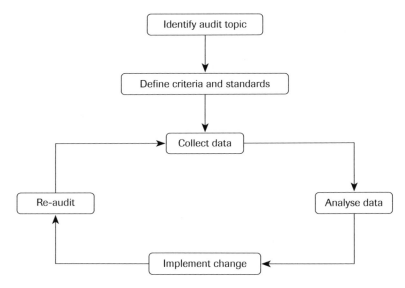

FIGURE 44.1 The audit cycle.

There are several approaches to clinical audit including:

➤ *Sentinel case audit*: examines variations from the norm in terms of outcome.

➤ *Random case-note review*: examines standards of note keeping and quality of administrative documentation.

➤ *Criterion-based review*: examines departures from specified criteria.

➤ *Outcome review*.

➤ *Patient satisfaction*: aims to improve service delivery.

AUDIT STANDARDS

➤ Need to reflect the special nature of healthcare of older people (atypical presentation, multiple pathologies, functional impairment and need for multidisciplinary assessment and treatment).

➤ Need to take account of national policy (NSF), good practice recommendations (NICE), as well as local professional and service experience in establishing principles.

➤ Standards need to be measurable, reflect success or failure of outcome and be locally determined on a multidisciplinary basis.

➤ The standards set should cover:
  — service organisation
  — service delivery
  — service evaluation
  — reflect the needs of the local population and not just the service
  — training, education and research.

➤ The Clinical Effectiveness and Evaluation Unit (CEEU) of the Royal College of Physicians aims to improve the quality of care delivered to patients in the National Health Service by ensuring that best practice and evidence-based approaches to care are widely disseminated and used for the benefit of patients. The activities of the CEEU include:

➤ The production of national clinical guidelines.

➤ The design of national comparative clinical audit tools to evaluate standards of organisation and delivery of clinical care.

➤ The coordination of national comparative clinical audit projects.

➤ The development of clinical outcome measures.

National audits of particular relevance:

➤ National Sentinel Audit of Stroke (Round 7 is due in 2010).

➤ The National Audit of Continence Care (next round in 2010).

➤ The National Clinical Audit of Falls and Bone Health in Older People (next round in 2010).

➤ National Sentinel Audit of Evidence-based Prescribing in Older People (EBPOP) (1999/2000).

➤ National Care of the Dying Audit of Hospitals (2008/2009).

CLINICAL GOVERNANCE

➤ Clinical governance is the framework through which NHS organisations are accountable for continuously improving the quality of their services and safeguarding high standards of care, by creating an environment in which clinical excellence can flourish.

➤ In order to be effective, standards must be measurable, achievable, relevant and acceptable.

➤ The establishment of national standards, supplemented by a system of inspection, has supported the development of a framework for clinical governance in the UK. The Care Quality Commission is responsible for inspection of standards in the NHS and independent sector in England.

➤ It should create an environment to monitor and detect whether a doctor's practice or care is of sufficient standard, and help identify those who are incompetent, dysfunctional or experiencing health problems which impair their practice.

➤ It improves the quality of care overall and highlights performance that deviates from the standards of quality and safety expected for a particular practice setting.

Five sectors of clinical governance have been identified:
➤ Clinical audit.
➤ Clinical effectiveness.
➤ Clinical risk management.
➤ Quality assurance.
➤ Staff and organisation development.

DEALING WITH COMPLAINTS
What is a complaint?
People will naturally have queries in relation to their care and treatment. Some will be expressed in conversation and others in writing. A query is generally viewed as a complaint if having had immediate action taken to resolve the concerns or the promise of a resolution, the complainant remains dissatisfied. The Citizen's Charter Complaints Task Force defined a complaint as 'an expression of dissatisfaction requiring a response'.
➤ All complaints, whether verbal or written, should receive a positive and full response in a timely fashion, with the aim of:
   — Satisfying the complainant that his/her concerns have been listened to.
   — Offering an apology where applicable.
   — Offering an explanation.
   — Showing that appropriate action has or will be taken.

Complainants want to make their views known in a climate, which is receptive and constructive. The Health Service Commissioner (Ombudsman) identified poor staff attitude as the single biggest cause of complaints being referred to him for investigation.

WHAT IS RELICENSURE?
At its present stage of development it is likely that relicensure will be subject to the following requirements:
➤ the doctor engaging in satisfactory annual appraisal
➤ participation in a workplace-based but independent 360-degree, or multi-source, feedback exercise
➤ resolution of concerns or issues about a doctor's conduct or practice, to the satisfaction of the medical director or responsible officer and the regional GMC.

APPRAISAL
➤ Appraisal is a systematic approach to review a person's achievements (linked to delivery of service and objectives), consider their continuing progress and to identify development needs.
➤ It is a retrospective review of professional activities with a prospective element and the development of a personal development plan (PDP).
➤ It is a recognised requirement for being a doctor and should be an annual process.
➤ It should contain a judgement on the person's performance against clear standards, and not just be a development guidance.
➤ It should take place in the context of, and be informed by, local clinical governance systems.
➤ It is confidential, and in its current format appraisal is not of itself a mechanism for picking up and addressing serious concerns. Other systems, including clinical governance, will need to be able to do this.
➤ Linked to clinical governance, it is likely to be the prime form of evidence required for licensing and revalidation. This is the process currently being developed by the GMC by which doctors will receive a license at 5-yearly intervals allowing them to continue to practise medicine in the UK.

FURTHER READING

Dickinson E, Sinclair AJ. Clinical audit of health care. In: MSJ Pathy, editor. *Principles and Practice of Geriatric Medicine*. Chichester: John Wiley & Sons; 1989.

General Medical Council. *Good Medical Practice*. London: General Medical Council; 2006.

Good Medical Practice. *A Working Framework for Appraisal and Assessment*. London: General Medical Council; 2008.

Royal College of Physicians. www.rcplondon.ac.uk

CHAPTER 45

NHS structure and management

- ➤ The NHS was launched in 1948.
- ➤ The largest publicly funded health service.
- ➤ Its core principle is that good healthcare should be available to all, irrespective of wealth. With the exception of some prescription charges, dental and optical services it remains free at the point of use for UK residents.
- ➤ The NHS is funded from national taxation and its current budget is more than £100 billion.

The NHS is controlled by the Department of Health, led by the Secretary of State for Health who works with five ministers of health, the NHS Chief Executive and the permanent secretary. The role of the Department of Health is to provide strategic leadership to the NHS and social care organisations. The department also has UK-wide responsibilities in areas such as international and EU business, licensing and safety of medicines, planning for pandemic flu, and so on. Within the Department of Health are clinical directors who oversee the implementation of clinical programmes such as the National Service Frameworks (NSFs). In 2007, responsibility for these clinical programmes was transferred to a new post of NHS Medical Director.

The Department of Health controls the 10 strategic health authorities (SHAs) in England, which in turn supervise all the NHS trusts (except foundation trusts) in their area. The devolved administrations of Scotland, Wales and Northern Ireland run their services separately and while there are some differences they remain similar in most respects. This chapter focuses on the NHS in England.

The SHAs are responsible for:
- ➤ Developing plans for improving health services in their local area that reflect national policy as well as local need.
- ➤ Ensuring local health services are of high quality and perform well financially.
- ➤ Workforce development including education, training and workforce planning.

Special health authorities were set up to provide a national service to the NHS or the public under the NHS Act 1977. They are independent but can be subject to ministerial direction. They include the National Institute for Health and Clinical Excellence (NICE), National Patient Safety Agency (NPSA) and the National Blood and Transplant Authority.

The NHS is divided into two sections: primary and secondary care.
- ➤ *Primary care* is the first point of contact for most people and is delivered by a number of independent contractors including GPs, dentists, pharmacists, opticians. NHS direct and NHS walk-in centres are part of primary care.
- ➤ *Primary care trusts* (PCTs) are in charge of primary care and commissioning secondary care. They work with local authorities and other agencies that provide

health and social care locally to ensure local needs are met. They are at the centre of the NHS and currently control 80% of the NHS budget. They have responsibility for developing practice-based commissioning, whereby general practices have their own budgets and are responsible for commissioning services that meet the needs of the local population.

➤ *Secondary care* includes emergency care and elective or planned specialist medical or surgical care and includes the following trusts:
  — *Acute trusts* are responsible for managing hospitals and also provide some community services through health centres, clinics or in people's homes. They ensure that hospitals provide high quality care and manage their finances efficiently. Some acute trusts are regional or national centres for specialised care and others are attached to universities and help train health professionals. The Department of Health expects that all NHS trusts will become foundation trusts in the near future.
  — *Foundation trusts* were introduced in 2004. They are NHS hospitals run by local managers, staff and members of the public and tailored to the needs of the local population. They are constituted as separate non-profit organisations and are owned by their members who are local people, employees and other key stakeholders. They have more financial and operational freedom than other NHS trusts but remain within the NHS and its performance and inspection system (Care Quality Commission). Monitor is the independent regulator that issues a licence for the foundation trust to operate and is responsible for ensuring that the terms of the licence are upheld.
  — *Ambulance trusts.* There are 12 ambulance services in England that provide emergency access to healthcare. Emergency calls for an ambulance are prioritised into life threatening and non-life threatening. In the former, a rapid response vehicle will be sent, crewed by a paramedic and equipped to provide treatment at the scene of an incident. In some areas the ambulance trust also provides transport to bring patients to hospital for treatment.
  — *Care trusts* provide both health and social care. The NHS and local authorities agree to work together to ensure a closer relationship between health and social care. At present they are few in number but more will be set up in the future.
  — *Mental health trusts* provide mental health and social care for people with mental health problems in England. Services may be provided by the GP, other primary care services or more specialist services and are overseen by the local PCT.

➤ *Trust management structure.* The management board of NHS and foundation trusts comprises a chief executive, director of finance and a number of non-executive directors. The management board has overall responsibility for the day-to-day management of the hospital and clinical services are managed through clinical directorates or similar-type structures.

OTHER NHS AND NON-NHS ORGANISATIONS

One of the aims of the current NHS reforms is to increase the capacity of the NHS by developing other types of NHS providers and allowing non-NHS providers to contract for services. The white paper on the future of community services – *Our Health, Our Care, Our Say* – requires that more care be provided closer to the patient's home. As a result, a number of organisations have developed that will be delivering healthcare in the future. These include:
➤ *Clinical Assessment, Treatment and Support services* (CATS) may be operated by the NHS or the independent sector. Referrals from general practitioners are assessed in these centres with the aim of reducing referrals to hospitals.

➤ *Treatment centres* are stand-alone organisations usually providing elective surgery and some diagnostics such as radiology and endoscopy. They may be run by the NHS but more typically these are operated by the independent sector.
➤ *Primary care centres* provide services such as out-patient clinics, urgent care (alternative to accident and emergency departments for non-trauma patients), renal dialysis, and endoscopy and may also include walk in centres that focus on emergency care.
➤ *Independent hospitals.* Increasingly, NHS patients are being referred to independent hospitals for NHS care such as elective surgery.
➤ *Polyclinics* include many of the services seen in a primary care centre but include general practitioners. They are currently been developed and it is likely that many of these clinics will be owned and run by the independent sector.
➤ *Social enterprise ventures and the Third Sector* are organisations that are run along business lines but profits are reinvested into the community or service developments. The Department of Health is encouraging the formation of these organisations with dedicated funding as a way of delivering innovative health and social care. Services provided include alcohol and substance misuse programmes, services for vulnerable adults, and other community-based services. They are part of the third sector, non-NHS, non-independent sector, including voluntary, non-profit organisations and charities.

DEVELOPMENT OF CLINICAL SERVICES

To ensure that the national priorities are implemented, a number of strategies have been developed which include:
➤ *National Service Frameworks* (NSFs) were launched in 1998. They set national standards, define the way a service should be provided and establish performance milestones against which progress can be measured with the aim of raising quality and decreasing variation in NHS services. There are nine NSFs to date including one for older people, published in 2001.
➤ *Priorities and Planning Framework.* The Department of Health increasingly focuses national priorities on a number of targets, which are updated annually. These targets (called 'vital signs') are set at three levels: Tier 1, must dos; Tier 2, national priorities for local delivery, e.g. abolition of mixed-sex accommodation, improving end of life care; and Tier 3, locally agreed targets. PCTs as commissioners of service need to ensure these targets are met.
➤ *NHS performance rating.* The Care Quality Commission was established in April 2009 and replaced three separate regulators for health, social services and mental health. All providers of healthcare must be registered with the Care Quality Commission who is responsible for carrying out the Annual Health Check. This is a published annual rating for each NHS organisation, based on performance in a number of areas, including performance against the Standards for Better Health and national targets and priorities. It includes clinical services and financial performance.
➤ *Quality contracts and quality accounts.* The review of the NHS in England carried out by Lord Darzi has led to a significant change in health policy in England, placing a greater emphasis on the quality of services, and all healthcare providers must now publish a quality account. Primary care trusts have to agree to a quality contract with the trust or provider. Through the Commissioning for Quality and Innovation payment framework (CQUIN) scheme, a proportion of the providers' income for a service is linked to quality and innovation.

FINANCING OF THE NHS IN ENGLAND

PCTs either on their own or through practice-based commissioning are responsible for commissioning services from NHS trusts, foundation trusts, independent hospitals or other non-NHS providers. Different systems operate in Scotland, Wales and Northern Ireland. The commissioning arrangement is through a nationally agreed contract, which specifies the number of cases to be treated, the quality standards (set by the Care Quality Commission) to be achieved and the price of the treatment, which is based on a national tariff price. The tariff is based on the average cost of a coded episode of patient care called a Healthcare Resource Group (HRG). Competition between providers is based on access, volume and quality of the services rather than the price. This system is called Payment by Results (PbR).

Another factor that influences the market is patient choice. When a GP decides a patient needs referral for treatment, the patient is offered a choice of hospitals (including independent hospitals and treatment centres, etc.) that provide the service and can then book the appointment electronically from the GP's surgery using the Choose and Book software.

FURTHER READING

Galloway M. *The ACP Guide to the Structure of the NHS in the United Kingdom*. Hove: Association of Clinical Pathologists; 2009.

Department of Health. *High Quality Care for All*. London: Department of Health; 2008.

Department of Health. *Using the Commissioning for Quality and Innovation (CQUIN) Payment Framework*. London: Department of Health; 2008.

Nicholson D. *High Quality Care for All: the operating framework for the NHS in England 2009/10*. London: Department of Health; 2008.

Department of Health. *Our Health, Our Care, Our Say*. London: Department of Health; 2006.

CHAPTER 46

NICE, HASCAS and NHS QIS

NATIONAL INSTITUTE FOR HEALTH AND CLINICAL EXCELLENCE (NICE)

NICE is an independent organisation responsible for providing national guidance on promoting good health and preventing and treating ill health. The three areas of health covered include:

➤ *public health*: promotion of good health and the prevention of ill health for those working in the NHS, local authorities and the wider public and voluntary sector
➤ *health technologies*: use of new and existing medicines, treatments and procedures within the NHS
➤ *clinical practice*: appropriate treatment and care of people with specific diseases and conditions within the NHS.

The Darzi report, *High Quality Care for All* (June 2008),[1] expanded NICE's role to include setting and approving more independent quality standards for the NHS, particularly with regard to:

➤ clinical effectiveness
➤ patient safety
➤ patient experience.

NICE Guidance

➤ Developed using the expertise of the NHS and the wider healthcare community including NHS staff, healthcare professionals and patients (through consultation and workshops).
➤ Developed by considering research studies about different types of treatment, interventions and care and how well they do or do not work.
➤ Balances the needs and wishes of individuals and the groups representing them, against those of the wider population. This sometimes means treatments are not recommended because they do not provide sufficient benefit to justify their cost.

To help its work NICE has specifically established:

➤ The Citizens Council made up of 30 members from the population in England and Wales to access the views of the public.
➤ The Partnership Council – members are nominated by groups representing patient and public interests, health professional bodies, academic institutions, NHS management, healthcare quality organisations, industry (companies producing drugs, devices and diagnostic equipment) and trade unions.

THE HEALTH AND SOCIAL CARE ADVISORY SERVICE (HASCAS)

➤ Started out as the Health Advisory Service (HAS) within the Department of Health (DoH) 40 years ago.
➤ In 1997, a consortium comprising the British Geriatrics Society, the Royal College of Psychiatry and the Office of Public Management took over responsibility from the DoH.
➤ In 2003, HAS merged with the Centre for Mental Health Services Development to form the Health and Social Care Advisory Service (HASCAS).
➤ Now a registered charity and a limited company.
➤ Provides independent advice and support to local organisations with an aim of improving services for older people across health and social care. Local organisations include:
    — healthcare trusts, i.e. PCTs, acute care trusts, mental health trusts
    — strategic health authorities
    — Department of Health
    — voluntary and public sector organisations
    — social service departments
    — local authorities.
➤ Workforce Development Confederations.

HASCAS can help develop specific solutions to local problems by:
    — defining a vision and strategy development
    — performing independent investigations
    — standards/practice development
    — service re-design
    — workforce planning
    — team development
    — development of community mental health teams (CMHTs) for older people
    — mentoring for managers
    — improving the dignity of care through workshops and audit tool.

Recently HASCAS has worked on behalf of the Department of Health to:
➤ Support primary care trusts (PCTs) develop and improve the quality of their intermediate care services for older people with mental health needs.
➤ Examine the quality of inpatient care in acute trusts for older people and the impact the inpatient experience itself had on timely discharge.
➤ Look at quality of life after a stroke.
➤ Develop and successfully run a number of outcome-orientated dignity workshops.

NHS QIS (NATIONAL HEALTH SERVICE QUALITY IMPROVEMENT SCOTLAND)

NHS QIS is an umbrella organisation for:
➤ The Scottish Health Council, which monitors NHS boards.
➤ The Scottish Intercollegiate Guidelines Network (SIGN), promoting consistence in clinical practice and clinical outcome.
➤ The Healthcare Environment Inspectorate: its remit is to inspect Scottish hospitals, ensuring the highest standards of infection prevention and cleanliness in order to help reduce infections within hospitals and raise public confidence.

NHS QIS:
➤ Takes a lead role in coordinating the work of the Scottish Patient Safety

Programme and provide support to the Scottish Medicines Consortium who advise on the clinical effectiveness and cost effectiveness of all newly-licensed medicines.

➤ Helps NHS Boards improve patient care by:
— providing advice, guidance and setting standards
— supporting implementation and improvement
— assessing, measuring and reporting the performance of NHS Board.

REFERENCE

1 Department of Health. *High Quality Care for All: NHS Next Stage Review final report*. London: Department of Health; 2008. Available at: www.dh.gov.uk/en/publicationsandstatistics/publications/publicationspolicyandguidance/DH_085825 (accessed 20 May 2010).

FURTHER INFORMATION

Health and Social Care Advisory Service www.hascas.org.uk
National Institute for Health and Clinical Excellence www.nice.org.uk
National Health Service Quality Improvement Scotland www.nhshealthquality.org

Index